Pesticides:
Health, Safety and the Environment

Pesticides:
Health, Safety and the Environment

G.A. Matthews

International Pesticides Application Research Centre
Imperial College
Silwood Park
Ascot, Berkshire
UK

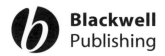

Blackwell
Publishing

© 2006 G.A. Matthews

Blackwell Publishing Ltd
Editorial Offices:
Blackwell Publishing Ltd, 9600 Garsington Road, Oxford OX4 2DQ, UK
    Tel: +44 (0)1865 776868
Blackwell Publishing Professional, 2121 State Avenue, Ames, Iowa 50014-8300, USA
Tel: +1 515 292 0140
Blackwell Publishing Asia Pty Ltd, 550 Swanston Street, Carlton, Victoria 3053, Australia
    Tel: +61 (0)3 8359 1011

First published 2006 by Blackwell Publishing Ltd

ISBN-13: 978-14051-3091-2
ISBN-10: 1-4051-3091-1

Library of Congress Cataloging-in-Publication Data
Matthews, G. A.
    Pesticides: health, safety, and the environment/G.A. Matthews.
        p. cm.
    Includes bibliographical references (p.   ) and index.
    ISBN-13: 978-1-4051-3091-2 (hardback: alk. paper)
    ISBN-10: 1-4051-3091-1 ((hardback: alk. paper)
    1. Pesticides. 2. Pesticides–Environmental aspects. 3. Pesticides
    –Health aspects. I. Title.
    SB951.M5127 2006
    632′ .95--dc22

                                                            2005032039

A catalogue record for this title is available from the British Library

Set in 10/11 pt Palatino
by Sparks, Oxford – www.sparks.co.uk
Printed and bound in India
by Replika Press Pvt, Ltd, Kundli

The publisher's policy is to use permanent paper from mills that operate a sustainable forestry policy, and which has been manufactured from pulp processed using acid-free and elementary chlorine-free practices. Furthermore, the publisher ensures that the text paper and cover board used have met acceptable environmental accreditation standards.

For further information on Blackwell Publishing, visit our website:
www.blackwellpublishing.com

Contents

Preface   vii
Acknowledgements   ix

1 Pesticides and agricultural development   **1**
   Principal pesticides   3
   Major crops   9
   Forests   15
   Tillage   15
   Amenity areas and home gardens   16
   Nuisance pests and vector control   16
   Legislation   16

2 Approval of pesticides   **29**
   Retrospective assessment   38
   Environmental aspects   40
   Endocrine disrupters   41
   Approval in relation to efficacy   43
   Operator proficiency   43
   Waste management   44

3 Application of pesticides   **46**
   Hydraulic sprayers   46
   Space treatment equipment   66
   Granule application   68
   Seed treatment   69
   Storage of pesticides and equipment   70
   Timing and number of spray applications   71

4 Operator exposure   **78**
   Methodology of measuring exposure   85
   Exposure of hands   88
   Inhalation exposure   91
   Biomonitoring   92
   First aid   94
   Periods of exposure   95

5   **Spray drift, bystander, resident and worker exposure**   **108**
      What is drift?   109
      How is drift measured?   110
      Airborne droplets   112
      Bystander exposure   115
      Residential exposure   120
      Worker exposure   126

6   **Environmental aspects of spray drift**   **133**
      Protecting water   133
      Protecting vegetation   147
      Protecting birds   151
      Overall environmental impact assessments   155

7   **Residues in food**   **168**

8   **The future of pesticides**   **184**
      Weed management   184
      Disease management   185
      Insect management   186
      Traditional plant breeding   187
      Present day pesticides   191
      Other insecticides   194
      More selective applications   196
      Pheromones   197
      GM crops   199
      Perceptions and hopes for the future   201

Appendix 1 – Some standard terms and abbreviations used in the
     approval of pesticides   207
Appendix 2 – Checklist of important actions for pesticide users   219
Appendix 3 – A note on the publication of the Royal Commission on
     Environmental Pollution Report and reply by the Advisory
     Committee on Pesticides   221
Index   223

Preface

Pesticides have undoubtedly helped to increase agricultural production and control vectors of disease over the past five decades, but there has been increasing criticism since Rachel Carson alerted users to the side effects of some pesticides in the environment. My own involvement dates back to before Rachel Carson's book *Silent Spring* as I was with a team of entomologists seeking to control insect pests of cotton in Africa. We recognised then that pesticides should only be used in conjunction with other control tactics, a system recognised in the USA and much publicised as integrated pest management. In the UK, authorities had also responded to early problems due to use of highly toxic pesticides and the adverse effects of birds due to organochlorine insecticides by establishing the voluntary Pesticides Safety Precaution Scheme. While developed countries introduced registration of pesticides, requiring detailed scientific data on which to base a risk analysis, many other countries did not have the resources needed to operate a detailed registration system. In consequence, highly toxic pesticides have been used in many countries, especially in tropical areas where protective clothing, as used in temperate climates, is unacceptably hot and uncomfortable to wear. This has led to many cases of illness and death following exposure to these highly toxic pesticides. These problems have been increasingly recognised and efforts made to harmonise registration requirements. This book sets out to emphasise that, apart from the correct choice of pesticide, it is the way it is applied that impacts on people, either directly on those using the many commercial products, but also others by the movement of pesticides in the environment and as residues in harvested produce.

Application technology has largely been ignored, and it has been left to engineers to design machinery that is easy to use and is as inexpensive as possible for the user. It is, however, a complex multidisciplinary subject which affects us all. Following the previous book *Pesticide Application Methods*, which dealt with the different equipment that can be used, this book explains how the registration process can avoid use of the pesticides that pose a significant risk to users and the environment, and how by a better understanding of the subsequent movement of pesticides following application, the risk of any adverse impact following their use can be minimised. Today, carefully applied pesticides, used only when needed, can contribute to higher productivity and allow us to feed and protect the growing human population. This requires much better education and practical training with certification so that pesticides are indeed applied more accurately and with greater safety than in the past. It is hoped that this compilation of data will help readers to have a better understanding of how pesticides can be applied without harming the users and adverse pollution of their environment. In addition, the overall management of pesticides, covering packaging, storage and proper stock control, needs to be improved so as to avoid having obsolete stocks of pesticides. Unfortunately, many countries still have obsolete pesticides that need careful disposal to avoid pollution of the environment.

There is a vast amount of information that has been published in scientific journals and books, so only selected data have been used in writing the chapters. More information is now available via the internet, not only from official web sites of government agencies and agrochemical companies but also from pressure groups. However, care is needed in choosing appropriate sources of information as sometimes only part of a story is reported. As with many complex subjects these days, it is important that as holistic approach as possible is taken to obtain the benefits of the technology while minimising adverse effects.

Graham Matthews
August 2005

Acknowledgements

I wish to thank the following, who have read and commented on one or more chapters and for supplying information: Roy Bateman, Tom Bals, David Buffin, John Clayton, Theodor Friedrich, John Furman, Richard Glass, Paul Hamey, Andrew Hewitt, Philippa Powell, Bill Taylor and Carol Ramsay. A special thank you also to Moira for her understanding and encouragement while I was writing this book.

I am also indebted to the following for the supply of photographs and other illustrations: Bill Basford, Roy Bateman, Central Science Laboratory, John Chandler (Exocet), Alison Craig (PAN UK), Vincent Fallon (whose photograph was supplied by Georgina Downs), Greg Doruchowski, Benedict Gove, Franklin Hall, Hans Ganzelmeier, Richard Garnett (Wisdom Systems), Hardi International, Professor Brian Hoskins (Reading University), Househam Sprayers, Kilgerm Chemicals, Kathy Lewis, Micron Sprayers Limited, Paul Miller (Silsoe Research Institute), Philippa Powell (Royal Commission on Environmental Pollution) and Jan Van der Zande.

1 Pesticides and agricultural development

Today, farmers regard pesticides as an essential tool to ensure that they can maintain production of crops of quality and quantity to satisfy an increasing human population. If we look back only some sixty years, farmers had to rely very much on crop rotations and mechanical weed control with hoes, hoping for a good dry spell of weather so that the weeds dried and were not merely moved. They also hoped that insect pests and disease control could be ameliorated by choosing a good crop variety, that had some resistance to pest damage. Cultural and biological control of pests were inadequate, so farmers needed a quicker and more reliable method of pest control. Recent estimates of crop losses due to insect pests, diseases caused by various pathogens and competition from weeds, despite present control practices, range from 26 to 40% for major crops, with weeds causing the highest potential loss (Oerke and Dehne, 2004).

Prior to 1940, some chemicals were available, notably the botanical insecticides, such as the pyrethrins, nicotine and rotenone (derris), but they were not widely used, largely because they deteriorated rapidly in sunlight. A few inorganic chemicals, notably copper sulphate, lime sulphur and lead arsenate, were also available. However, it was the development of synthetic organic pesticides during and following World War II that revolutionised the control of pests. Chemists had been looking for a cheap chemical with persistence in sunlight and low toxicity to man that would kill insect pests quickly, and in 1938 Muller showed that DDT would indeed fit this specification. Its availability during World War II led to initial use as a 10% dust on humans, for example in Naples, to suppress a typhus outbreak (Crauford-Benson, 1946). Soon afterwards it became available for agricultural use and began to be applied extensively on crops, such as cotton, at rates up to 4 kg ai/ha. Its use has had a major impact on vector control, being responsible, for example in India, for reducing the annual death rate due to malaria from 750,000 to 1500 during the first eight years it was applied. Recognition of problems associated with the persistence of DDT in the environment were only realised later and highlighted by Rachel Carson in her book *Silent Spring* (Carson, 1962).

Parallel with the new insecticides, the development of 2,4-D as a herbicide controlling broad-leaf weeds in cereal crops made a similar major impact on

Table 1.1   Year of introduction of selected pesticides (Ware, 1986; Tomlin, 2000)

Year	Pesticide type	Pesticide
1850	Herbicide	ferrous sulphate
1882	Fungicide	Bordeaux mixture
1930	Herbicide	DNOC
1931	Fungicide	thiram
1939	Insecticide	DDT (commercialised 1944)
1942	Herbicide	2,4-D
1943	Fungicide	zineb
1944	Insecticide	HCH (lindane)
1946	Insecticide	parathion
1948	Insecticide	aldrin, dieldrin
1949	Fungicide	captan
1952	Insecticide	diazinon
1953	Herbicide	mecoprop
1955	Herbicide	paraquat (commercialised 1962)
1956	Insecticide	carbaryl
1965	Nematicide	aldicarb
1968	Fungicide	benomyl
1971	Herbicide	glyphosate
1972	Insecticide	diflubenzuron
1973	Insecticide	permethrin
1990	Insecticide	imidacloprid
	Fungicide	azoxystrobin
	Insecticide	spinosad

agriculture. While copper fungicides had been available since the end of the nineteenth Century (Lodeman, 1896), further research has led to a greater range of more selective fungicides. These discoveries (Table 1.1) led to a rapid development of many other pesticides over the following decades. *The Pesticide Manual* is one important source of information on currently manufactured pesticides. Individual countries have lists of products that are registered for use. In the UK, this is published as *The UK Pesticide Guide*. Information can be obtained also from a number of internet sites. Using a search engine such as Google, information relevant to the UK is available through the Pesticides Safety Directorate web page, while the Environmental Protection Agency provides similar information in the USA. The Pesticide Action Network and many universities also have web pages with pesticide information.

In Western Europe and North America the availability of herbicides was a major breakthrough at a time when shortages of labour due to the world war, industrialisation and urbanisation all played a part in necessitating a change in weed management on farms. Spraying fields with a herbicide allowed the crop seeds to germinate and to develop without competition from weeds, thus increasing the yield potential that could then also benefit from fertiliser applications. The discovery of paraquat, a herbicide that killed

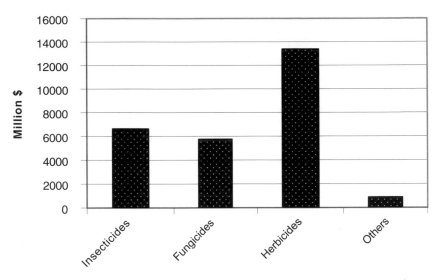

Fig. 1.1   World sales of pesticides, 2003.

all weeds, enabled a new concept of minimum or zero-tillage to reduce the need for ploughing fields every year and thus reduce the risk of soil erosion in many areas of the world. The more recent herbicide glyphosate is now likely to be used more extensively with the advent of herbicide-tolerant, genetically modified crops.

The availability of a wider range of chemicals and international marketing of pesticides has led to a global growth in their use. Total global sales of pesticides had declined slightly in 2002 to approximately $25 million per annum, but had increased again in 2003 to $26.71 million. This is composed of almost 50% herbicides, 25% insecticides and 21.6% fungicides, and the remainder to other products (Fig. 1.1). Most pesticides are used in North America, which accounts for about one-third, with Western Europe and East Asia accounting for one-fifth each, and Latin America the next largest market (Fig. 1.2). The above data are based on marketing statistics, as few countries have survey data on the actual usage of pesticides. Thomas (2000) describes the system operated in the UK to obtain accurate and timely information to satisfy government legislation. The data are also helpful in relation to the registration process and review of approved products.

Principal pesticides

The following sections provide a brief account of some of the pesticides now available.

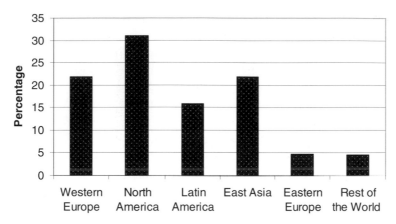

Fig. 1.2   Global sales of pesticides by region.

Insecticides

Initially the two main types of insecticides were the organochlorine (OC) and organophosphates (OPs), both being neurotoxins – that is, they affect the nervous system. The OC insecticides, including DDT, dieldrin and endrin, had one main advantage, namely their persistence that enabled farmers to achieve control over a long period. However, plant growth and rainfall reduced the effectiveness of deposits on foliage. Later it was realised that this attribute led to residues remaining in the environment and being accumulated in some animals at the end of food chains. In consequence, these chemicals can be found everywhere, although their use has now been banned, except for endosulfan (although it will not be accepted on Annex 1 of Directive 91/414/EEC in Europe) and DDT, the latter being used on a limited scale in vector control.

Organophosphate insecticides are a diverse group (Anon, 1999), some of which are extremely toxic (e.g. parathion, methidathion and monocrotophos), while others, such as temephos, malathion and trichlorfon, are much less hazardous to use. When used in place of the OC insecticides, more people suffered acute poisoning, as the need for protective clothing had not been adequately recognised in many countries. Many people now consider that those classified as the most hazardous to use (see later) should also be banned. In the UK, most of these highly hazardous chemicals were not approved, although a few, such as chlorfenvinphos and chlorpyrifos, were registered for control of specific pests. Other OPs, such as diazinon, have been used extensively in sheep dips. Karalliedde *et al.* (2001) provide a critical overview of organophosphates and their impact on health.

Another group with a similar mode of action is the carbamates, though these also vary very much in their toxicity. The most toxic examples, including aldicarb and carbofuran, were only allowed registration in the UK as granules and not as sprays, to reduce potential exposure. The less-toxic carbaryl has been very widely used as a broad-spectrum insecticide. Newer insecticide groups include the pyrethroids and neonicotinoids.

Natural pyrethrins extracted from dried flower heads of *Chrysanthemum cinerariaefolium* had been known for centuries as a potent insecticide, but they were rapidly inactivated, when exposed to sunlight. Efforts at Rothamsted Experimental Station in the UK (now Rothamsted Research) led to the development of synthetic photostable pyrethroids, permethrin, cypermethrin and deltamethrin (Elliott *et al.*, 1973; Elliott *et al.*, 1978). Other pyrethroids have been developed, so this group became the most popular broad-spectrum insecticide group.

More recently, the neonicotinoids, notably imidacloprid, have been rapidly accepted, especially where insects are resistant to the earlier types of insecticide. A feature of these newer chemicals and fipronil, a phenylpyrazole, is that they are active at extremely low dosages.

In contrast to the nerve poisons, insect growth regulators, such as diflubenzuron, affect insect development, mostly by adversely affecting chitin synthesis so the insect fails to complete a moult from one larval stage to the next. Another novel insecticide, tebufenozide, causes larvae to form precocious adults; that is, they attempt to moult into an adult before sufficient larval development has taken place.

There is now greater interest in the development of natural organisms such as the fungus *Metarhizium anisopliae* as a biopesticide, a strain of which is very effective against locusts and other acridids. One advantage is that they are selective, but this presents difficulties in marketing a product that is effective against only a limited number of pests. Entomopathogenic nematodes have also increased in importance to control certain pests that attack plant roots such as the vine weevil. Biopesticides also tend to be slower acting, but they do integrate well with other biological control agents.

Herbicides

Herbicides are the most extensively used group of pesticides, except by small-scale farmers in Third World countries. Already their use is a crucial part of mechanised farming in North America, Europe and Australia. However, many small farms have great difficulty in coping with weed control at the critical stages of early crop establishment. This is accentuated in areas where disease, such as HIV/Aids, has reduced the number of people available for weeding and people have migrated to cities.

Herbicides can act on *contact* with a plant or are *translocated* within the plant. Good spray coverage is needed with contact herbicides. Sometimes only part of the foliage is affected so some weeds, although adversely affected, will survive. Translocated herbicides are important for many different weeds, but are particularly important for controlling perennial weeds, such as some of the key grass weeds. An example of a translocated herbicide is glyphosate, which will move down into the rhizomes of grasses, rather than only affect the foliage above ground. As the herbicide is distributed within the plant, good coverage is slightly less important.

Herbicides can also be classified according to the time of application. Weed control may be by means of *preplanting* application. This is usually a soil treatment that affects weed seeds before the crop is sown. After the crop has been sown, a *pre-emergence* herbicide will selectively affect the weed species without interfering with the germination and growth of the crop. When farmers have to contend with erratic rainfall and are not sure if a crop can be established, they may opt for a *post-emergence* herbicide applied later to the weeds. The herbicide may be applied to the whole of the crop area, or in the case of post-emergence herbicides, the spray can be applied as a band in the inter-row, or in some cases along the intra-row, using mechanical cultivation of the inter-row. The latter technique is useful with crops that have been genetically modified to be resistant to particular herbicides that can be sprayed over the crop. In contrast, where a crop may be very sensitive to the herbicide, sprays need to be directed to avoid contact with the crop. Individual clumps of weeds can be spot-treated, or if certain weeds are confined to specific areas of a field, the farmer can carry out patch spraying.

Herbicides may be broad spectrum, affecting all types of weeds, or they may be selective. In most cases, selectivity is between monocotyledon weeds (e.g. grasses) and dicotyledons, the broad-leaved plants. There are many different groups of herbicides, based on their chemical structure. The Weed Science Society of America has provided a classification of herbicides. A few important groups are mentioned here. Most have a very low mammalian toxicity. Most concern regarding human toxicity has been directed at paraquat, as it is lethal if the concentrated liquid reaches the lungs. A detailed assessment of paraquat poisoning has been reported by Lock and Wilks (2001).

Aryloxyphenoxy propionates

These have good activity against grass weeds in broad-leaf crops as a post-emergence translocated herbicide. One example is fluazifop-butyl.

Bipyridyliums

Paraquat is the most important in this group. It damages foliage quickly on contact, but is also very strongly adsorbed onto the soil and rendered ineffective. The rapid wilting and desiccation of foliage within hours has enabled effective weed control to be achieved in many crops, where the spray is directed away from the actual crop. It has been extensively used in tree crops, such as rubber plantations.

Dinitroanilines

Trifluralin is a good example of a pre-planting soil-incorporated herbicide to reduce the impact of grass weeds in a broad-leaf crop. Low water solubility minimises leaching and movement within the soil, but being volatile they must be covered by the soil.

Phenoxy or 'hormone' herbicides

2,4-D and MCPA are highly selective for broad-leaf weeds, being translocated throughout the plant, affecting cellular division.

Phosphono amino acids

Glyphosate and glufosinate are foliar-applied, translocated herbicides that interfere with normal plant amino acid synthesis. They are non-selective, but more effective against grasses than broad-leaf weeds. There is no soil activity. They are formulated to improve uptake by the plants as rainfall shortly after application can reduce effectiveness.

Substituted ureas

Most of these, such as isoproturon, flumeturon, diuron and linuron, are non-selective, pre-emergence herbicides, which are absorbed in the soil and then taken up by roots. Some are active as foliar-applied, post-emergence herbicides.

Sulfonylureas

This is a large group that is used mainly to control broad-leaf weeds by inhibiting meristematic growth. Metsulfuron-methyl and others in the group have both foliar and soil activity and are active at extremely low application rates – a few grams per hectare. However, if small amounts remain active in the soil too long, the following crop may be affected.

Triazines

This group includes one of the most used herbicides, atrazine, which was very effective as a post-emergence spray in maize. However, it has been implicated in environmental problems, as it has been claimed that very low doses in water have an endocrine disruption effect that has resulted in a decline in frog populations, so it has been withdrawn from certain uses.

Table 1.2   Some examples of fungicides

Type of fungicide	Example
Triazoles	propiconazole
	tebuconazole
Morpholines	fenpropimorph
Anilinopyrimidines	cyprodinil
Benzimidazoles	carbendazim
Carboxamides	carboxin [only in mixtures]
Strobilurins	azoxystrobin
Others	chlorothanil

Fungicides

The use of sulphur to protect vines dates back to ancient Greek civilisations, and with Bordeaux mixture since the end of the nineteenth century, most developments of fungicides have occurred only in the past few decades. Apart from the contact, protectant fungicides, such as copper fungicides and mancozeb, a number of systemic fungicides (see Table 1.2) with different modes of action have been developed (Hewitt, 1998), most recently the stobilurins. Unfortunately, pathogens that are susceptible to a particular type of fungicide often become less sensitive. Thus, great care is needed to avoid selection of pathogens resistant to a fungicide, by only applying those with a particular mode of action for a short period before using a different type in rotation. Manufacturers have also recommended mixtures as a means of delaying selection of resistant strains. Fungicidal seed treatments are important to protect young seedlings.

Rodenticides

Significant crop losses can be caused by rodents, both in the field and in stores. Rats are also a major problem in cities and other areas where they can obtain food. Various poisons have been set out in baits, usually inside traps to prevent other mammals (especially dogs) from gaining access to the poison. Following the use of the anti-coagulant warfarin, to which rats have become resistant, other rodenticides such as bromadiolone and difenacoum have been introduced. There is particular concern that predatory birds can be affected by eating rodents that have consumed a poisoned bait, but have not yet died.

Crop distribution

The distribution of pesticide use by crop is illustrated in Figure 1.3. Public concern is directed mainly at the amounts of insecticides and fungicides used on food crops, especially those that are eaten without further processing.

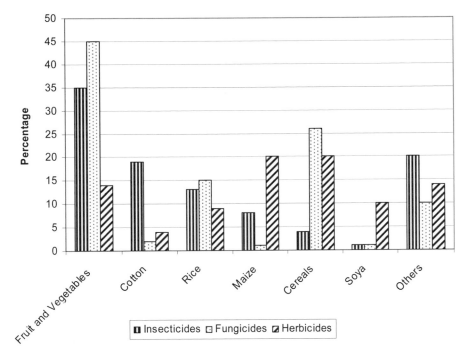

Fig. 1.3   Global sales of pesticides by major crops.

Major crops

The application of pesticides has been an important component of changes in agricultural practices, including new crop varieties that have enabled yields of major crops to be increased. While they have not increased the yield potential, they have enabled farmers to realise a higher proportion of the potential yields by reducing the losses due to pests and pathogens and from weed competition. In addition, improved quality of the harvested produce has allowed longer storage under suitable conditions that enables marketing of the crop to be extended. A few examples of the higher yields harvested are shown below.

Wheat

Yields of wheat worldwide average only 2.6 t/ha, although the potential is much higher as shown by the improvement in yields achieved in the UK (Table 1.3). Much of the yield benefit in the UK has been due to efficient weed management following the introduction of herbicides. A return to the days of manual weeding is unthinkable as the cost of labour would be too high. In the UK, with organic agriculture, the estimate for casual labour for some vegetable crops can be as much as 40 days per hectare at £5.70 per

Table 1.3   Area and yield of wheat in the United Kingdom

Year	c.1932	1969–71	1971–81	1988–90	1999	2003
Area harvested (1000 hectares)	980	1434	1994	1847	1837	
Yield (mt/ha)	2.1	4.2	5.6	8.8	8.0	7.8

hour, although mechanical hoeing would be done where possible to avoid manual weeding.

In California, a state law was enacted to ban weeding crops with short-handled hoes as the work was excessively arduous, but use of long-handled hoes was considered to cause some crop damage.

Rice

Success with breeding new high-yielding varieties of the 'Green Revolution' in Asia led to higher yields and production (Table 1.4), but led to increased pest problems. Use of insecticides is generally blamed for the outbreaks of the brown planthopper, *Nilapavata lugens*, as insecticides were promoted in some areas as if they were like fertilisers to increase yields. In practice, the poor application of broad-spectrum insecticides made the planthopper problem worse as little spray reached the lower part of the stem favoured by the nymphs. The pest problem was also due to the overlapping of two or more rice crops, with little attention given to a closed season between harvesting and sowing a second crop. Improvements in variety selection, which enables farmers to sow resistant varieties, has reduced the planthopper problem and by avoiding any insecticide use during the first six weeks of plant development, natural enemies have been able to exert adequate control of most pests (Way and Heong, 1994). Farmer field schools, promoted by the Food and Agriculture Organization (FAO), have been more effective in lowland-irrigated rice areas as the system was based on extensive research at the International Rice Research Institute (Matteson, 2000). One of the problems in adopting integrated pest management (IPM) is getting farmers to accept that crop losses are not always as high as they perceive (Escalada and Heong, 2004).

Table 1.4   Yields of rice (t/ha rough rice) from http://www.irri.org/science/ricestat/pdfs

Year	Global	China	India	Japan
1962	1.89	2.08	1.54	5.14
1972	2.32	3.25	1.60	5.85
1982	2.98	4.89	1.85	5.69
1992	3.59	5.90	2.61	6.28
2002	3.92	6.27	2.91	6.63

However, rice farmers also have to contend with weeds as the increased cost of labour has resulted in changes from the transplanting of seedlings to more extensive use of direct seeding. Yield losses as high as 46% caused by weeds have been reported, so in some areas, farmer adoption of herbicides has increased rapidly during the past decade, although alternative crop establishment methods have also been adopted to reduce weed problems. Crops may need to be sprayed with fungicide in some areas due to diseases, such as rice blast.

Cotton

In many cotton-growing areas of the world, insect pests have been a major constraint on production. The discovery that DDT was effective against the bollworm *Helicoverpa zea* in the USA and *H. armigera* in the Old World enabled farmers to more than double their yields. Instead of yields of less than 500 kg seed cotton per hectare, obtained when the crop was grown 'organically', farmers could expect to get over 1000 kg/ha (Tunstall and Matthews, 1966; Gower and Matthews, 1971) (Fig. 1.4), and with good rainfall or irrigation much higher yields are possible with the variety best suited to local climatic conditions. However, in many countries heavy insecticide use soon led to other problems by eliminating the natural enemies of other insects feeding on cotton plants; thus, the boll weevil (*Anthonomus grandis*) became the major problem in the USA. Escalation of insecticide use occurred with mixtures of insecticides, such as DDT + methyl parathion + toxaphene, and higher

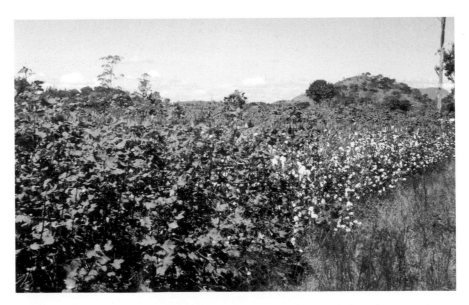

Fig. 1.4 Contrast between untreated cotton with many insect pests and sprayed cotton with crop ready for harvesting in Malawi (photograph GAM).

dosages were applied until the selection of pests resistant to the insecticides became very evident. The situation in cotton has now changed with the introduction of genetically modified cotton (see Chapter 8) that has already led to fewer insecticides sprays needed against bollworms.

Maize

Intensive production of maize with pesticide inputs allows yields of over 9 t/ha, whereas farmers in many areas of Africa barely produce 0.5 t/ha. The major problem is initially weeds, which are highly competitive with young seedlings during the first three weeks after seed germination. Traditionally, African farmers have hoed their crops (Fig. 1.5), but the amount of time and effort needed often results in part of the sown area being abandoned. No doubt a major weed *Striga* will be tackled using a maize resistant to a herbicide applied as a seed treatment. Locusts, armyworms and stem borers (Fig. 1.6) can also decimate young maize crops. Whereas locusts and armyworms tend to be sporadic pests, stem borers are a chronic problem, which can be controlled by a relative small amount of insecticide, provided it is in the whorl of leaves of the young plants (Fig. 1.7), although much effort is now being put into breeding Bt maize which is resistant to lepidopteran pests. Crop protection is again crucial when the grain is harvested.

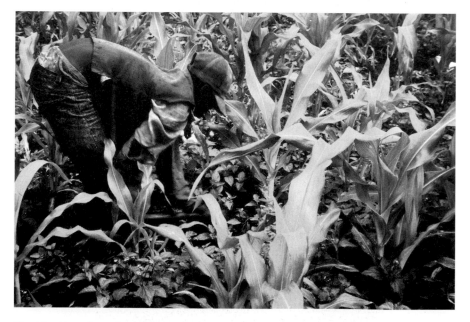

Fig. 1.5   Manual weeding of maize.

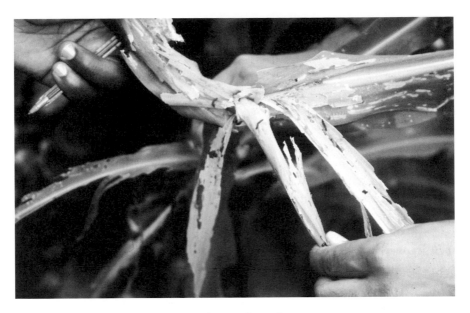

Fig. 1.6 Maize damaged by stem borer (photograph GAM).

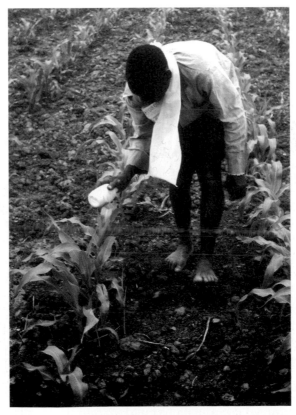

Fig. 1.7 Simple granule treatment with insecticide to control stem borers (GM maize with the Bt gene could eliminate the need for this inexpensive treatment, but seed will be more expensive) (photograph GAM).

Fruit
Bananas

A major disease of the 'Cavendish' variety (which accounts for about 10% of global production) of bananas, Sigatoka, has resulted in growers resorting to fungicide applications, usually applied by aircraft on large estates. A new form of the disease, black sigatoka, and a new strain of fusarium wilt, also known as Panama disease, are causing particular concern, as these are far less easy to control. Bananas, with plantains, are widely grown on small farms in Africa, largely for local consumption, but a major drop in production in Uganda occurred due to failure of disease control in 1980, plus nematode and banana weevils. Some farmers are now growing new resistant varieties imported from Central America. Meanwhile, a major effort is underway to develop new disease-resistant varieties.

Apples

Apart from a number of insect pests, such as the codling moth, apple orchards can suffer from mildew and scab diseases. Much emphasis has been placed on controlling insects with pheromone traps and encouraging natural enemies, but several fungicides sprays may be needed during the season. In the UK, research is aimed at endeavouring to control the pathogen late in the season after harvesting in order to reduce the carry-over of infection to the following season. Fewer early-season fungicide sprays should then control the disease and also reduce the likelihood of any pesticide residues in the apples.

Vegetables
Potatoes

Commercial yields of potatoes vary from around 18 to over 45 tonnes per hectare depending on the variety and soil type, but also on protection from nematodes, late blight and insect pests. In the UK, the average yield is about 45 t/ha, but the plants may be sprayed as many as 13 times during the season. If untreated, late blight, which was the cause of the Irish famine (1846–50), can spread very rapidly with as much as 75% of foliage destroyed in less than 10 days. In fungicide trials yield increases of up to 30 t/ha have been reported. Similar devastating crop damage can also be inflicted by the Colorado beetle (*Leptinotarsa decemlineata*), which has spread from the USA across Europe to Asia. Yield loss due to viruses transmitted by aphids is usually low in the year in which the crop acquires infection, but if those tubers are used as seed potatoes, the yield will decline rapidly. Thus, farmers obtain certified seed potatoes from areas with low aphid infestations. However, aphids may still need to be controlled if populations build up rapidly. Ideally, crop rotation is used to minimise nematode damage, but nematicides are still required where potatoes are grown one year in four on the same land.

Tomatoes

In the tropics, tomatoes are grown in fields, but in Mediterranean and temperate climates the crop is in plastic or glasshouses. Yields as high as 200 t/ha have been harvested, but protection from pests and diseases is essential. In a more controlled environment, the trend has been away from using insecticides to greater reliance on biological control, but protection from several diseases is still essential.

Forests

Certain insect pests can cause major defoliation of large areas of forests. In North America, the spruce budworm (*Choristoneura fumiferana*) and the gypsy moth (*Lymantria dispar*) are among the key pests that have led authorities to spray large areas with insecticides. In the early days of these programmes, broad-spectrum insecticides were used, but currently *Bacillus thuringiensis* (Bt), a biological pesticide and other more ecological acceptable products are sprayed. In Poland, control of the nun moth (*Lymantria monacha*) was achieved over 2.5 million hectares using aerially applied Bt and the chitin inhibitor, diflubenzuron in 1994–7. Thus, control operations are crucial in some years to preserve forests.

Tillage

Farmers have for centuries used crop rotation and traditional tillage by ploughing and hoeing to manage weeds in the fields. However, in some parts of the world, ploughing may adversely affect earthworms, while the loosening of the soil makes it prone to erosion. There is, therefore, awareness that for some crops reducing tillage – usually referred to as conservation tillage – has certain advantages. The aim is to protect the soil from the damaging effects of rain splash by leaving 30–50% stover on the soil surface. This should then reduce run-off and retain more rain on the fields. Various techniques have been developed to sow and plant the crop, for example by using a narrow furrow or just individual planting holes. Most of the land is undisturbed, but with the lack of burying weed seeds, conservation tillage does depend on careful use of herbicides to avoid weed competition. This is an area in which greater use of herbicides offsets the costs of using less tillage.

Amenity areas and home gardens

Significant quantities of pesticides are now used by local authorities, for example in keeping pathways and drains free of weeds. More emphasis has been given to non-chemical methods where these are effective, but cost-effective treatments are required, as several chemicals have been banned due to the contamination of water supplies. A limited number of pesticides are now marketed for home and garden use, notably for controlling insect pests on tomatoes, roses and lawns. In the UK, only those considered to be safe to use without professional training, and those that do not require the use of any protective clothing, are permitted. Many of these products have been sold in ready-to-use forms in small plastic containers incorporating a trigger-operated nozzle.

Nuisance pests and vector control

The control of ants and cockroaches in dwellings was often carried out by applying a low concentration dust to areas where the insects are known to live. The alternative has been to use pressure packs, known more usually as aerosol cans. Professional operators controlling nuisance pests in restaurants, hospitals, aircraft and other locations use a range of different spray equipment. On a larger scale, where the control of mosquitoes has required urban action, vehicle-mounted cold fogging equipment or aircraft may be used to apply insecticide at the flight time of the mosquitoes. Mosquito control units are present in most counties throughout the USA, and these have been particularly active following the outbreak of West Nile Virus.

Legislation

Right from the outset concerns were raised about the use of some of these new chemicals. In some countries, such as Germany, legislation demanded the registration of pesticides with the Federal Institute of Biology for Agriculture and Forestry (BBA). Regulation of pesticides in the USA began as long ago as 1910, but in 1972 the Federal Insecticide, Fungicide and Rodenticide Act was developed from a labelling law and now regulates the manufacture, distribution and use of pesticides. In contrast, in the UK, for many years there was a voluntary scheme – the Pesticides Safety Precautions Scheme – alongside an Agricultural Chemicals Approval Scheme established by the pesticide industry with the government health and agricultural authorities. In 1985 The Food and Environment Protection Act brought the UK into line with changes within Europe, so that the registration of pesticides became a statutory requirement. Subsequently, various regulations, which are periodically amended, form part of the overall Act. These include the Control of Pesticides Regulations (COPR) 1986, the Maximum Residue Levels in (Crops, Food and Feeding Stuffs) Regulations 1994 and the Control of Substances Hazardous to Health (COSHH) Regulations. Alongside the Act there are Statutory Codes of Practice. More information on legislation is given in Chapter 2.

In Europe, the Council of the European Union has established new legislation that controls the registration of plant protection products under Directive 91/414.EEC. When an active ingredient is approved at EU level, it is placed on Annex 1 and may be used by member states. However, commercial formulations of pesticides still require registration in individual countries. Requirements for registration are discussed in Chapter 2. In the international sphere, the FAO has sought to achieve harmonisation of the data requirements since the *Ad Hoc* Government Consultation on Pesticides in Agriculture and Public Health (FAO, 1975). Following this meeting, the FAO published a Code of Conduct, which has been subsequently amended and now includes the requirements for Prior Informed Consent (PIC) aimed at assisting the less-developed countries without the resources to administer a full registration system to decide whether it should allow the import of certain pesticides. The FAO Code now has incorporated the FAO Minimum Requirements for Application equipment.

The World Health Organization (WHO) has published a classification system (Table 1.5) for pesticides, based on the acute toxicity of the formulation. Class I pesticides are the most hazardous to use, whereas those in the unclassified category are the least toxic to mammals. The examples in Table 1.6 show that Class I pesticides are mostly the older types of insecticides. The Codex Alimentarius Commission of the United Nations is responsible for harmonisation of standards related to the international food trade and by collaboration with the Joint meetings of a FAO Working Party and a WHO Expert Committee, the Codex Committee on Pesticide Residues sets international standards. The International Union of Pure and Applied Chemistry (IUPAC) also has a role in setting specifications for each pesticide.

Table 1.5   WHO Classification (http://www.who.int/ipcs/publications/en/pesticides_hazard.pdf)

Class	Hazard level	Oral toxicity[#]		Dermal toxicity[#]	
		Solids*	Liquids*	Solids*	Liquids*
Ia	Extremely hazardous	<5	<20	<10	<40
Ib	Highly hazardous	5–50	20–200	10–100	40–400
II	Moderately hazardous	50–500	200–2000	100–1000	400–4000
III	Slightly hazardous	>500	>2000	>1000	>4000
U	Unclassified				

[#]Based on LD_{50} for the rat (mg/kg body weight).
*The terms 'solids' and 'liquids' refer to the physical state of the product or formulation being classified.

Table 1.6   Examples of pesticides according to WHO Classification in relation to mammalian toxicity for the active substance. The type and concentration of the formulation will adjust the ranking, thus pyrethroid insecticides are used at a low concentration, so considered less hazardous

Class	Insecticide	Fungicide	Herbicide	Rodenticide
Ia	aldicarb mevinphos parathion phorate phosphamidon	captafol		brodifacoum
Ib	azinphosmethyl carbofuran dichlorvos formetanate metamidophos methomyl monocrotophos nicotine triazophos			warfarin
II	bendiocarb carbosulfan chlorpyrifos cypermethrn deltamethrin dimethoate fenitrothion fenthion fipronil imidacloprid lambda cyhalothrin rotenone thiodicarb	azaconazole copper sulphate fentin hydroxide tetraconazole	2,4-D paraquat	
III	acephate amitraz malathion resmethrin spinosad trichlorfon	copper hydroxide copper oxychloride metalaxyl thiram	ametryn bentazone dicamba dichlorprop glufosinate isoproturon linuron MCPA mecoprop propanil	
Unclassified	phenothrin temephos	axoxystrobin benomyl carbendazim iprodione mancozeb sulphur	atrazine glyphosate simazine trifluralin	

The agrochemical industry has grown over the past 50 years, accompanied by increasingly vociferous opposition to the use of pesticides. In some areas of the world an increased incidence of problems of human health is associated with lack of regulation, and this has resulted in the most toxic insecticides being used by illiterate farmers, usually without training or adequate protection during their application (Fig. 1.8). Estimates of poisoning cases are not easy in many countries with a poor infrastructure. In some countries, many affected by poisoning may not see a doctor and only a small proportion reach a hospital for proper treatment. In 1972, the WHO estimated from 19 countries that as many as 500,000 cases of poisoning occurred each year (WHO, 1973), with a later estimate suggesting about 20,000 deaths a year due to pesticides (Anon, 1990; Forget *et al.*, 1993).

The most horrific number of deaths was at Bhopal in India in 1984, when a chemical methyl isocyanate (MIC) used at a factory making the carbamate

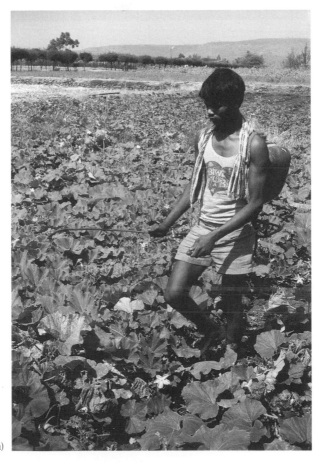

(a)

Fig. 1.8 Contrasts in protective clothing while using a lever-operated knapsack sprayer. (a) India (photograph GAM). (*Continued.*)

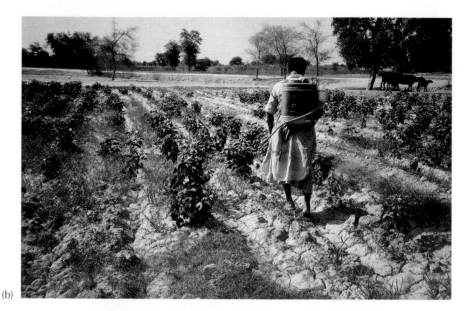

(b)

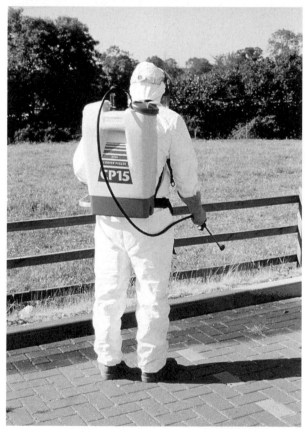

(c)

Fig 1.8   (*Continued.*) (b) Pakistan (photograph GAM); (c) United Kingdom (photograph Hardi International). (*Continued.*)

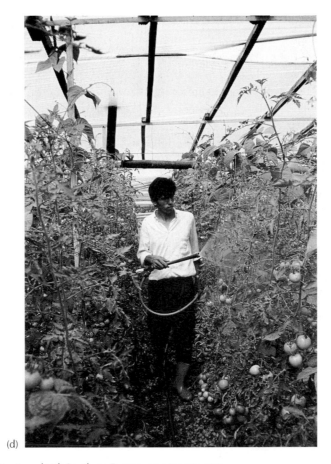

(d)

Fig 1.8 (*Continued.*) (d) Southern Europe, on a tomato crop.

insecticide carbaryl (Sevin) was contaminated with water. The reaction led to an extremely toxic gas escaping and this killed over 4000 people in the following hours. Regrettably, vast numbers had been allowed to live in slums close to the factory, and with no contingency plans these people were not protected from the toxic gas. Even more were affected by the gas and suffered severe health problems. Some estimates indicate as many as 15,000 died later, with many more continuing to suffer from chronic symptoms.

In the Soviet Union, there was rapid expansion in the use of pesticides, so that by the 1980s the USSR was one of the world leaders in pesticide use in terms of per hectare and per capita. Unfortunately, the pesticides were often of inferior quality, packaged in large containers, poorly stored and inefficiently applied, often by aircraft. This led to vast numbers of people being poisoned, with for example the average daily concentration of OPs such as demeton over 0.1 mg/m^3 in air, at distances of 500–1000 m from the cotton fields (Fedorov and Yablokov, 2004). This extensive poisoning in Uzbekistan led to a switch to biological control and the setting up of biofactories to produce parasitoids. This practice is still adopted in the country, although some use of pesticides is needed with diversification of their agriculture.

Reports have shown that the US Military sprayed 42 million litres of a mixture of herbicides known as Agent Orange to defoliate large areas, and this caused the world's largest dioxin contamination in South Vietnam between August 1961 and April 1971. Possible birth defects caused by exposure to this mixture led to the sprays being discontinued, but it has left a long-term legacy of environmental and health effects, which are still being investigated (Palmer, 2005). Levels of the dioxin TCDD in soil, food and human samples remain elevated in areas, where Agent Orange had been applied by low-flying aircraft and in areas where spillages occurred from stores at military bases (Dwernychuk *et al.*, 2002). Later in 1976, an explosion at a chemical plant in Seveso, Italy, exposed residents over an area of 18.1 km^2 to an aerosol cloud with the highest exposure of TCDD known in humans. Numerous animals died, and 193 cases of chloracne were reported among the residents (Eskenazi *et al.*, 2001).

Globally, the cause and symptoms of poisoning vary between chemicals and countries (Harris, 2000). In some cases, where deaths have occurred, it is undoubtedly due to application of pesticides classified by WHO as Ia or Ib pesticides, with no protective clothing being worn. Some of the OP insecticides, such as parathion, methamidophos and monocrotophos, were used more when application of organochlorine insecticides was discouraged and because farmers perceived that these killed their pests quickly. In some countries deliberate drinking of pesticides in suicide attempts has been the main cause of death, rather than occupational exposure.

In Sri Lanka, the total national number of admissions due to poisoning doubled between 1986 and 2000, with an increase in admissions due to pesticide poisoning of over 50%, though the number of deaths fell. In particular, the number of deaths due to the OP insecticides, monocrotophos and methamidophos, fell from 72% of pesticide-induced deaths as the import was restricted and eventually banned in 1995 However, the use of these insecticides was replaced by endosulfan (WHO Class II) and this led to a rise in deaths from one in 1994 to 50 in 1998 when this insecticide was also banned. Over the decade the number of deaths due to pesticide poisoning had not changed significantly, with WHO Class II OP insecticides becoming a major factor. The switching from one pesticide to another, especially in relation to self-poisoning, needs further attention and although legislation on pesticides had an effect, the emphasis now must be on other strategies to reduce the availability of the most hazardous chemicals (Roberts *et al.*, 2003; Konradsen *et al.*, 2003).

In China, there has been a major increase in the use of agricultural chemicals, including Class 1 OP insecticides, and unfortunately many fatalities have been reported. In Zhejiang Province, from 1997–2002, 1910 people died out of a total of 19,547 reported cases with pesticide poisoning. Of these cases,

3202 occurred as a result of occupational poisoning, and 23 of the patients died; all of the others were non-occupational poisoning (Lin *et al.*, 2004).

Sherwood *et al.* (2005) also reported considerable problems in one area of South America where operators are often heavily exposed to the highly toxic insecticides, such as carbofuran and methamidophos, and also suffer from dermatitis after the extensive use of fungicides. These two anti-cholinesterase insecticides and monochrotophos were the primary pesticides involved in pesticide poisoning in the rural populations of certain regions of the state of Mato Grosso do Sul (Recena *et al.*, 2005).

In South Africa, early indications are that smallholders, who adopted the growing of Bt cotton had a reduced incidence of skin disorders, feeling generally unwell, and other health effects that had been associated with spraying for bollworm. It has been suggested that if all farmers grew Bt cotton, the number of poisonings would decrease to just two per season, compared to 51 reported cases in the 1997–98 season (Bennett *et al.*, 2003). Similar reports have also come from China (Hossain *et al.*, 2004).

Unfortunately, in contrast to demands for the banning of many pesticides, less attention has been given to equipment, and the farmers have been left to choose and maintain their sprayers. In consequence, often cheap (e.g. <$10) and poorly maintained sprayers are used and this has frequently resulted in prolonged exposure to pesticides during spraying, by those who have poor facilities to wash after work. This is probably the cause of many cases of poisoning, especially with insecticide sprays. In order to prevent leakage of pesticide from the sprayer tank over the operator's body or leakage over unprotected hands, the FAO has published guidelines and minimum standards for pesticide application equipment (Anon, 2001).

In contrast to the developing countries, relatively few cases of acute poisoning are reported in temperate climates, where protective clothing is available and worn. The USA is the largest market for herbicides using paraquat, yet poisoning due to this herbicide is uncommon, with calls to US poison centres indicating only about 0.01% of reported cases involving paraquat or diquat (Hall, 1995), with almost no fatalities.

As most of the recorded fatalities have been due to suicidal ingestion of paraquat concentrate, the problem of accidental ingestion led the principal manufacturer of paraquat to introduce formulation changes to the liquid concentrate during the late 1970s and early 1980s (Sabapathy, 1995). A blue colour was added to prevent confusion with drinks, a stenching agent was introduced to alert users, and an emetic was included. In addition, packaging and labelling have been improved to prevent decanting of the product. Stewardship with emphasis on education and training has been directed in particular towards smallholder farmers in developing countries, where the majority of incidents occurred.

In the UK, the use of extremely hazardous pesticides is not allowed, except for a few nematicides, such as aldicarb, which are applied as solid granules to soil. Many other pesticides have now been withdrawn, either because the commercial company did not consider sales justified the cost of the additional test data needed to meet the current requirements of the EU, or additional data and evaluation has led to revocation of registration.

At the same time, led by the supermarkets, there has been a continued demand for 'organic' produce, ideally completely free of farmer-applied chemicals (a few chemicals have been permitted on organic crops), with various non-governmental organisations (NGOs) lobbying for pesticide reduction policies. Among the NGOs, the Pesticide Action Network (PAN) has sought to eliminate the hazards of pesticides, reduce dependence on them and prevent unnecessary expansion of their use, while increasing sustainable and ecological alternatives to chemical pest control (for example see Pretty, 2005). In response, the EU is developing a thematic strategy under which member states will have a national pesticide strategy. The aim will be to ensure sustainable crop production while minimising pesticide use.

However, in the USA and some European countries, the presence of pesticide residues in food has already led to a demand for pesticide-reduction policies. In some countries, this has been a policy of 50% reduction within a particular period of years. The question is then, a reduction of what? It is quite easy to reduce the quantity applied when a more active molecule, applied at a few grams per hectare, can be applied instead of an older product. Reducing the dosage of an application may be possible if it is correctly applied at the optimum time, but this is not always possible due to weather conditions. Some countries have also introduced targets to reduce the numbers of applications. However, the policy has encouraged the need for research into alternative strategies of pest control and emphasised a need for integrating different control tactics. Some governments have considered adding a tax on pesticides to reduce their use, but this is liable to increase costs of food when politicians favour keeping the cost of key foods as low as possible.

In the UK, in response to the threat of a pesticides tax, the Crop Protection Association introduced a Voluntary Initiative (VI) aimed at improving the standards of pesticide use through research, training, stewardship and communication. The success of this initiative is to be assessed by 18 indicators (see Chapter 6; some are listed in Table 1.7) that cover the protection of water (a 30% reduction in the frequency of detection of individual pesticides in untreated surface water at levels above 0.5 and 0.1 ppb), benefits to biodiversity by adoption of crop protection management programmes and changes in the behaviour of farmers through training. Best Practice Guides have now been distributed by Industry as part of the VI.

A parliamentary committee report in 2005 felt that the targets set by the VI were insufficiently challenging, but the scheme should continue after April 2006 with more focus on catchment-sensitive farming and other water issues. Members of the committee felt that much more study was needed to

Table 1.7   Some of the indicators covered by the Voluntary Initiative in the United Kingdom

Indicator	Target (by 31 March of year*)		
	31 Mar 2004	31 Mar 2005	31 Mar 2006
BETA qualified agronomists	100	400	750
Farm Environmental Management – Crop Protection Certificate qualified farmers	100	500	1250
Environmental Information sheets published	250	450	550 (estimate)
Crop Protection Management Plan area (ha)	200,000 (5% arable area)	900,000 (22.5% arable area)	1,200,000 (30% arable area)
National Register of Sprayer Operators (NRoSo) Members	15,000 (60% arable area)	17,500 (70% arable area)	17,500 (70% arable area)
Half Day Operator Roadshow events	90	120	150
Number of revised product labels	Not possible at this time to predict	All professional pesticides marketed by CPA members.	As 2004/5
Active agronomists on Professional Register (CPA distributor staff only)	100% compliance	As 2003/4	As 2003/4
National Sprayer Testing Scheme (NSTS) Tests	5,000 (20% arable area)	10,000 (50% arable area)	20,900 (80% arable area)

*Most of the Voluntary Initiative targets which relate to changing behaviour or which act as surrogates coincide with the Voluntary Initiative year. This runs from 1 April to 31 March.

examine the possibilities of a pesticide tax, since unless any revenue from this tax was returned to pay for pesticide mitigation action, it would merely have an adverse effect on farmers and be unjust. The schemes for sprayer testing and operator registration were welcomed, and it was considered that these should be mandatory, together with more action on the use of pesticides in amenity areas (Anon, 2005).

In addition to the VI, the UK Department of Environment, Food and Rural Affairs (DEFRA) had two public consultations in 2003. The first was to obtain views on the introduction of a no-spray 'buffer' between fields and residential properties, while the second was concerned with improving public access to information on the use of pesticides. Following these consultations, the Minister requested the Royal Commission on Environmental Pollution to report on the science used to assess the risk to people (bystanders and residents in areas close to farms) from crop spraying. The Commission examined a number of questions related to biological effects of pesticides on humans, the basis for assessing exposure to pesticides, legal aspects and government policy. In the UK, anyone who was concerned that they were affected by pesticides could report the incident and this was then examined by the Pesticide Incidents Appraisal Panel (PIAP). However, this scheme really only covered acute effects, so many people have argued that more attention should be paid to chronic effects, especially for those living close to agricultural land that was treated several times a year. Many have claimed that their ill-health was due to exposure to low concentrations of chemicals, leading to multiple chemical sensitivity syndrome (MCS), or they had reported chronic fatigue syndrome (CFS). Unfortunately, it is often extremely difficult to associate individual health problems with precise exposure data, but the Royal Commission considered that further research is needed using epidemiological studies and innovative methods, such as nuclear magnetic resonance (NMR) spectroscopy to investigate whether pesticide exposure is linked with chronic and multisystem illness. Recognising that many changes in the usage of pesticides have taken place, the Commission also recommended further assessment of exposure using probabilistic modelling validated by experimental data and various measures to reduce exposure. Furthermore, a National Pesticide Strategy should provide emphasis on the health of the public.

This chapter has shown that, despite the advantages farmers have gained from the availability of pesticides, numerous problems have arisen. In the following chapters, the way in which governments need to regulate their use is described and ways in which we can protect people are suggested.

References

Anon (1990) *Public Health Impact of Pesticides Used in Agriculture*. WHO, Geneva.

Anon (1999) *Organophosphates*. Committee on Toxicity of Chemicals in Food, Consumer products and the Environment. Department of Health, London.

Anon (2001) *Guidelines on Minimum Requirements for Agricultural Pesticide Application Equipment*. FAO, Rome.

Anon (2005) *Progress on the use of Pesticides: The Voluntary Initiative*. House of Commons: Environment, Food and Rural Affairs Committee Eighth Report of session 2004–2005.

Bennett, R., Buthelezi, T.J. Ismael, Y. and Morse, S. (2003) Bt cotton, pesticides labour and health: A case study of smallholder farmers in the Makhathini Flats, Republic of South Africa. *Outlook on Agriculture* **32,** 123–128.

Carson, R. (1962) *Silent Spring*. Hamish Hamilton.

Crauford-Benson, H.J. (1946) Naples typhus epidemic 1943–4. *British Medical Journal* **1,** 579–680.

Dwernychuk, L.W., Cau, H.D., Hatfield, C.T., Boivin, T.G., Hung, T.M., Dung, P.T. and Thai, N.D. (2002) Dioxin reservoirs in southern Viet Nam – A legacy of Agent Orange. *Chemosphere* **47**, 117–137.

Elliott, M., Farnham, A.W., Janes, N.F. Needham, P.H. and Pulman, D.A. (1973) Potent pyrethroid insecticides from modified cyclopropane acids. *Nature Lond.* **244**, 456.

Elliott, M., Janes, N.F. and Potter, C. (1978) The future of pyrethroids in insect control. *Annual Review of Entomology* **23**, 443–469.

Escalada, M.M. and Heong, K.L. (2004) A participatory exercise for modifying rice farmers' beliefs and practices in stem borer loss assessment. *Crop Protection* **23**, 11–17.

Eskenazi, B., Mocarelli, P., Warner, M., Samuels, S., Needham, L., Patterson, D., Brambilla, P., Gerthoux, P.M., Turner, W., Casalini, S., Cazzaniga, M. and Chee, W.-Y. (2001) Seveso Women's Health Study: Does zone of residence predict individual TCDD exposure? *Chemosphere* **43**, 937–942.

FAO (1975) *Report of* Ad Hoc *Government Consultation on Pesticides in Agriculture and Public Health.*

Fedorov, L.A. and Yablokov, A.V. (2004) *Pesticides: The chemical weapon that kills life (The USSR's Tragic Experience).* Pensoft, Sofia-Moscow.

Forget, G., Goodman, T. and de Villiers, A. (eds.) (1993) *Impact of Pesticide Use on Health in Developing Countries.* International Development Research Centre, Ottawa.

Gower, J. and Matthews, G.A. (1971) Cotton development in the Southern Region of Malawi. *Cotton Growing Review* **48**, 2–18.

Hall, A.H. (1995) Paraquat and diquat exposures reported to US Poison Centers 1983–1992. In: Bismuth, C. and Hall, A.H. (eds.) *Paraquat Poisoning.* Pp. 53–63, Marcel Dekker Inc., New York.

Harris, J. (2000) *Chemical Pesticide Markets, Health Risks and Residues.* Biopesticides Series 1, CABI Publishing, Wallingford.

Hewitt, H.G. (1998) *Fungicides in Crop Protection.* CAB International, Wallingford.

Hossain, F., Pray, C.E., Lu, Y., Huang, J. and Fan C. (2004) Genetically modified cotton and farmers' health in China. *International Journal of Occupational and Environmental Health* **10**, 296–303.

Karalliedde, L., Feldman, S., Henry, J. and Marrs, T. (eds.) (2001) *Organophosphates and Health.* IC Press, London.

Konradsen, F., van der Hoek, W., Cole, D.C., Hutchinson, G., Daisley, H., Singh, S. and Eddleston, M. (2003) Reducing acute poisoning in developing countries – options for restricting the availability of pesticides. *Toxicology* **192**, 249–261.

Lin, J., Yang, J., Ma, Z. and Sun, Y. (2004) Epidemiological analysis for pesticide poisoning in Zhejiang Province. *Zhejiang Prev. Med.* **16**, 7–10.

Lock, E.A. and Wilks, M.F. (2001) Paraquat. In: Krieger, R.I. (ed.), *Handbook of Pesticide Toxicology,* 2nd edn. Pp. 1559–1603, Academic Press, San Diego.

Lodeman, E.G. (l896) *The Spraying of Plants.* Macmillan, London.

Matteson, P.C. (2000) Insect pest management in tropical Asian irrigated rice. *Annual Review of Entomology* **45**, 549–574.

Oerke, E.-C. and Dehne, H.-W. (2004) Safeguarding production – losses in major crops and the role of crop protection. *Crop Protection* **23**, 275–285.

Palmer, M.G. (2005) The legacy of agent orange: empirical evidence from central Vietnam. *Social Science and Medicine* **60**, 1061–1070.

Pretty, J. (ed.) (2005) *The Pesticide Detox.* Earthscan, London.

Recena, M.C.P., Pires, D.X. and Caldas, E.D. (2005) *Acute Poisoning with Pesticides in the State of Mato Grosso do Sul, Brazil. Science of the Total Environment* (E-pub).

Roberts, D.M., Buckley, N.A., Manuweera, G. and Eddleston, M. (2003) Influence of pesticide regulation on acute poisoning death in Sri Lanka. *Bulletin of the WHO* **81**, 789–798.

Sabapathy, N.N. (1995) Paraquat formulation and safety management. In: Bismuth, C. and Hall, A.H. (eds.) *Paraquat Poisoning.* Marcel Dekker Inc., New York, pp. 335–347.

Sherwood, S., Cole, D., Crissman, C. and Paredes M. (2005) From pesticides to people: Improving ecosystem health in Northern Andes. In Pretty, J. (ed.). *The Pesticide Detox.* Earthscan, London, pp. 147–164.

Thomas, M.R. (2000) Pesticide usage monitoring in the United Kingdom. *Annals of Occupational Hygiene* **45**, S87–S93.

Tomlin, C.D.S. (2000) *The Pesticide Manual*. BCPC Publications.

Tunstall, J.P. and Matthews, G.A. (1966) Large scale spraying trials for the control of cotton insect pests in Central Africa. *Empire Cotton Growing Review* **43**(3), 121–139.

Ware, G.W. (1986) *The Pesticide Book*. Thomson Publications.

Way, M.J. and Heong, K.L.(1994) The role of biodiversity in the dynamics and management of insect pests of tropical irrigated rice. *Bulletin of Entomological Research* **84**, 567–587.

WHO (1973) *Safe Use of Pesticides*: Twentieth report of the WHO Expert Committee on Insecticides. Geneva, WHO Technical Report Series 513.

2 Approval of pesticides

Each pesticide has several names. As the chemical name (which is decided by the rules of the International Union of Pure and Applied Chemistry; IUPAC) is often long and complicated, pesticides are assigned a common name for the active ingredient agreed by the International Organisation for Standardisation (ISO). This pesticidal ingredient is used in one of more formulated products with trade names, which are regulated by marketing companies under national legislation. However, before they can be marketed, the companies developing pesticides must produce a large dossier of information to the regulatory authorities in the countries where they plan to market their products. In the USA, this is the Environmental Protection Agency (EPA). Changes in the European Union due to Directive 91/414/EEC, have resulted in the requirement for registration of the active ingredient to be completed initially before individual member states can register products/formulations containing the pesticide. One of the member states acts as the Rapporteur for compiling the assessment of the data to the EU committee.

In the UK, the Pesticides Safety Directorate (PSD), an executive agency of the Department of Environment, Food and Rural Affairs (DEFRA) is responsible for agrochemicals and links with the Health and Safety Executive in terms of products intended for other non-agricultural uses, known as biocides, such as treatment of timber, under The Biocides Directive (98/8/EEC) (Anon, 2000). Advice is provided by an independent expert committee, the Advisory Committee on Pesticides (ACP). This committee was set up following initial concern about the toxicity of the new pesticides during the 1940s and early 1950s on the recommendation of a Working Party on Precautionary Measures against Toxic Chemicals, set up in 1950, with Professor Zuckerman as chairman. In 1954, the Advisory Committee on Poisonous Substances used in Agriculture and Food Storage (ACPS) covered both pesticides and veterinary medicines used on farms. Veterinary medicines were removed from the committee's role after the Medicines Act in 1968, and since 1983 membership of the committee has been independent of both the Government and industry. Under the Nolan Rules, applicants are interviewed and those that meet the criteria in terms of specialist technical experience needed on the committee are short-listed for approval by the Minister. Recommendations made by the ACP go the Ministers, that is the Secretaries of State for Environment (with the Health and Safety aspects under the Department for Work and Pensions), Health, the Scottish Parliament and the Welsh Assembly, who must all agree on any decisions. Advice from the ACP is also used in Northern Ireland. The Royal Commission on Environmental Pollution has expressed concern that policy and regulation of pesticides is within one part of DEFRA and have recommended separation of these functions.

Pesticides are only approved if they are effective and cause no serious illness through their use, or harm anyone as a result of the level of residues in food or drinking water that might be found following Good Agricultural Practice (GAP). Furthermore, they should not cause any adverse effects to the environment when used according to the conditions of their approval. In order to meet these requirements, the data package is scrutinised in detail and a risk assessment made. The experimental work and preparation of the data package costs $150 million in health and environmental R&D.

In the UK, the companies can obtain an experimental approval to allow development studies on new pesticides, or new uses for existing pesticides, on a limited scale so that the scientific data on its efficacy and the residues obtained in treated crops can be determined. Unless the risk to consumers is assessed, the crop may have to be destroyed. A product may then be given provisional approval, which allows commercial use while additional confirmatory data that may be needed are obtained. Provisional approval is not granted, if there are outstanding 'safety' concerns.

Provisional approval under COPR in the UK is not the same as provisional authorisation under 91/414, for which all the data should be provided.

At present this level of approval also allows sales while the active ingredient is being evaluated under the new European system. In Europe, the European Food Safety Authority (EFSA) also performs a risk assessment, while risk management is carried out by the Health and Consumer Protection DG. There is also the Pesticide Risk Assessment Peer Review group and the Panel on plant health, plant protection products and their residues (PPR) at EFSA. Full approval for 10 years or longer is only given for a product when all the data requirements have been met and its use is assessed as not likely to harm human health or the environment

A product may be revoked if new evidence is obtained that, in commercial use, there are questions about its safety. The approval may also be reviewed if data requirements are changed. Many older products have been withdrawn recently because of more up-to-date data requirements and the manufacturers have not considered it financially cost-effective to invest in further research to support continued registration. The EU has acknowledged that some unsupported pesticides would be very unlikely to meet health and environmental standards, even if the money was spent on further safety testing.

On some occasions a product registered in one European country may be required in a different country. This is covered by a process of Mutual Recognition (MR), which allows for the harmonisation of product authorisations between member states (MS). This is only possible if it can be shown that the agricultural, plant health and environmental (including climatic) conditions relating to the use of the product are comparable in the regions concerned. On some occasions if a new alien pest is detected in the UK, special control measures may be needed to prevent its spread. This may require an emergency approval for a product not normally used in the UK, or approved only on certain crops.

Pesticides are poisons, and so a key aspect of the risk assessment is the potential toxicity to humans. Risk is a function of toxicity and exposure, so there can be a greater risk from a moderately toxic pesticide to which a person is highly exposed compared with a highly toxic pesticide but little exposure. In the UK the most highly toxic insecticides have not been approved for use as sprays, but some have approval used as granules. Much of the data required (Table 2.1) are obtained by experiments using the rat as a model mammal, but a few tests may be performed with dogs or rabbits. The number of laboratory animals used in these tests is kept as low as possible. Additional tests may be required depending on the mode of action of the pesticide and whether any effects on specific body systems, such as the nervous, immune or endocrine systems, need to studied in greater detail.

Table 2.1 Data requirements

Data type	Requirements
Metabolism	It is important to know what happens to the pesticide in the body, what metabolite(s) is (are) produced, and how it (they) is (are) excreted.
Acute toxicity	The effect of a single dose of the active ingredient and of the product by oral, dermal and inhalation exposure.
Chronic/'sub-acute' toxicity	The effect of exposure of the active ingredient when administered to animals over a long period. This test is usually for 2 years with rats, but a 1-year test may be needed with dogs.
Carcinogenicity	Whether the active ingredient has the potential to cause cancer when administered for a minimum of 2 years to rats, or 18 months to mice. Usually, data for two species are required.
Genotoxicity	Assessments of the potential of the active ingredient to damage the genetic material in cells.
Teratogenicity	Whether the active ingredient can cause fetal death or malformations when administered to female animals during pregnancy.
Generation study	In relation to chronic toxicity, has the active ingredient a potential to impair fertility and the ability to rear young?
Irritancy	Tests are also carried out to assess whether, when the active ingredient is applied, it will cause irritation to the skin or eyes, or has the potential to cause sensitisation, such as skin allergies. The outcome of these tests will affect the labelling of the product.

The long-term studies at a range of doses will indicate the feeding rate at which the active ingredient in milligrams per kilogram bodyweight (mg/kg bw) shows the first signs of any change in the test animals compared with untreated controls. Close observation will reveal any changes, apart from ill-health, that occur. Weight measurements are routine to see if there is any gain or loss. The tests will enable a dose, which defines the reference point below which no adverse symptoms occur. This is called the No Observed Adverse Effect Level (NOAEL). Sometimes reference is made to a No Observed Effect Level (NOEL) (Fig. 2.1).

This reference point is then used as a starting point to derive an acceptable daily intake (ADI), which is the amount of chemical that can be consumed every day for a lifetime in the practical certainty, on the basis of known facts, that no harm will result. In calculating safe daily intakes of food by humans, a 100-fold safety or uncertainty factor has been long established to allow for differences between the animal used in tests and humans and the inter-individual variability (Renwick *et al.*, 2000). Thus, it assumes that a human may be 10-fold more sensitive than a test animal, and a sensitive adult or child will be 10-fold more sensitive than the average human. These long-term tests take into account not only the active ingredient ingested, but also any metabolites produced in the body, as these may in some cases be more toxic than the original pesticide.

Concern about the so-called 'cocktail effect' of residues of more than one pesticide being found in a food sample has also been expressed. This aspect

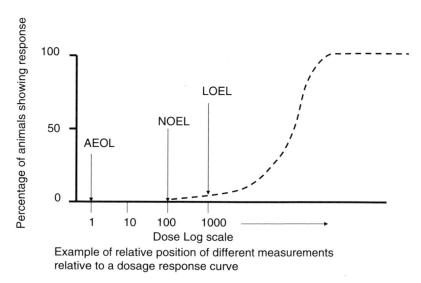

Example of relative position of different measurements relative to a dosage response curve

Fig. 2.1   Relative position of AEOL, NOEL and LOEL on a dosage response curve (Royal Commission on Environmental Pollution).

has been assessed in the UK by a committee set up by the Food Standards Agency. The Agency concluded that the risk to people's health from mixtures of residues is likely to be small. Although it considered that children and pregnant or breastfeeding women were unlikely to be more affected by the 'cocktail effect' than most other people, it was difficult, with only limited evidence, to predict how some chemicals would interact. Further research is needed, but in the interim the default assumptions for regulatory purposes are that chemicals with different modes of action will act independently and those with the same toxic action will act additively. Where there is a possibility of an interaction, such as potentiation, adequate dose–response data are essential for interpreting dietary intake and human exposure to the mixture (Woods, 2004).

On some days, people may consume much higher levels of certain foods or they may eat some foods only at one time in the year. In view of this, another important parameter is the Acute Reference Dose (ARfD). While similar to the ADI, it refers to the consumption of the amount of active ingredient at one meal or on one day. Short-term dietary intake was discussed by Hamilton *et al.* (2004), who reported the recommendations of the IUPAC Advisory Committee on Crop Protection Chemistry relating to acute dietary exposure. The value of ARfD is based on the lowest NOAEL obtained in acute toxicity or developmental toxicity tests, adjusted by an appropriate uncertainty factor. Guidance on setting the ARfD has been provided by Solecki *et al.* (2005).

The ADI and ARfD both relate to ingestion of the pesticide, whereas it is the skin of those working with pesticides that is often most exposed to the active agent. For these workers, the Acceptable Operator Exposure Level (AOEL) (Fig. 2.1) is the most important reference. The AOEL is set at a level of daily exposure that would not cause adverse effects in those working with the pesticide regularly over a period of days, weeks or months. It is calculated on the basis usually of short-term toxicity studies, usually of up to three months' duration, but other studies may be taken into account depending on the type of chemical and pattern of usage of the pesticide. Much of the emphasis on toxicology is related to the oral route, so numerous assumptions are made in worker risk assessments. It has been suggested therefore that methods of assessing dermal absorption, including the use of human subjects, need to be improved and that more needs to be known about interspecies pharmacokinetics to determine an appropriate toxicology study regime to reflect intermittent worker exposure (Ross *et al.*, 2001).

Information on pesticides, including the acute oral, dermal and inhalation toxicity, the NOEL, ADI, WHO toxicity class and EC hazard index is available from *The Pesticide Manual*, a publication of the British Crop Production Council (BCPC), that is also available in electronic format. Information on the registration of pesticides is provided in the UK for agricultural use by the Pesticides Safety Directorate (PSD), an agency of the Department of the Environment, Food and Rural Affairs (DEFRA), and by the Health and Safety Executive (HSE) for non-agricultural uses. A Guide is published that lists the active ingredients, which may be used on crops, and the pests controlled. This UK Pesticide Guide then provides a list of all products that have been registered for each active ingredient that has approval, and for each active ingredient, it lists the uses permitted, environmental safety, health classification and safety precautions required. An electronic version allows access to updates between the annual publication of the guide. Similar information is provided by all countries, which have a regulatory system. Further information is also available from the internet (e.g. http://www.epa.gov/pesticides; http://www.pesticideinfo.org; http://www.pesticides.gov.uk).

Before information reaches the ACP it is considered by an Inter-departmental Secretariat (IDS) formed by members of the UK regulatory departments, who also consider data being submitted under the European review programme under Directive 91/414.

The ACP also draws on the specialist knowledge of members of several other committees and panels that cover toxicology, the environment, residues and usage surveys. Minutes of ACP meetings are made available on the UK Pesticide Safety Directorate web page.

While the developed countries have appropriate legislation and government staff to implement the registration of pesticides, this situation does not exist on the same scale in developing countries. Some countries may have only a limited staff and virtually no support, such as residues laboratories. These countries have tended to rely on whether a pesticide has been registered by the EPA or in a European country.

Some have introduced local labelling requirements such as colour coding to indicate the WHO classification. Thus, in Zimbabwe, pesticides had to have a purple, red, orange or green label according to whether the product was in WHO Class I, II, III or unclassified, respectively. In order to buy purple- or red-labelled products, which were not openly displayed by distributors, the purchaser had to ask specifically for them and was required to know about the higher toxicity of the pesticide. In Brazil, pesticides are now purchased through an approved 'agronomist' – rather like having a prescription to obtain pharmaceutical products from a chemist.

Responsible registration of pesticides has limited the use of the most toxic pesticides in many countries, or has restricted their use to fully trained operators. In contrast, a lack of enforced regulation in many other areas of the world has allowed untrained people access to highly toxic pesticides. Doctors in developing countries have had to deal with many cases of poisoning as a result of highly toxic insecticides being applied without adequate protective clothing (Ngowi *et al.*, 2001). Unfortunately, many deaths caused by pesticides are the result of suicides, where people have over-used the pesticide and then had insufficient income from their crop to repay debts. This has been particularly noted in parts of Asia.

One of the main causes of pesticide poisoning among farmers in the tropics is exposure to the concentrated formulated product when preparing sprays. Measuring out small quantities of pesticide to apply with manually operated equipment exposes the operator's hands, unless suitable packaging such as sachets (Fig. 2.2) is used or farmers are provided with ancillary equipment to allow the safe measurement of small quantities. Subsequently, the spray operator is exposed to the diluted spray while walking through crops, and improved coveralls are needed that are suitable for hot climates and will protect areas of the skin, such as the lower legs, which are most exposed to a spray. Spray operator training and certification will need to be increased, but this is a major task in tropical countries with very many small farms.

Clearly, with an increasing world population to be fed, pesticides will continue to be an important tool in integrated pest management/integrated crop management (IPM/ICM) (see Chapter 8) programmes, but for this to be more acceptable greater efforts are needed to minimise ill health due to operator exposure as well as minimising environmental pollution.

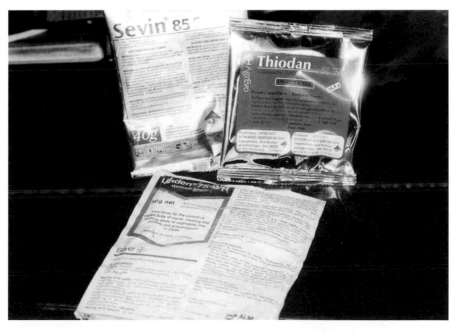

(a)

Fig. 2.2   Different containers. (a) Sachets. (*Continued.*)

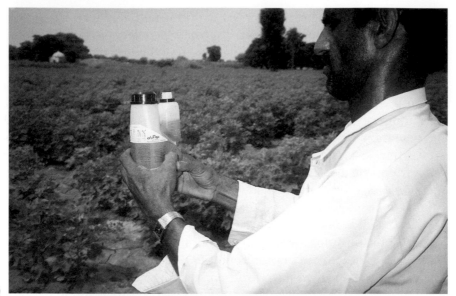

(b)

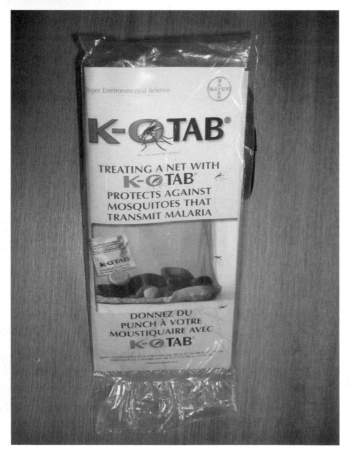

(c)

Fig. 2.2   (*Continued.*) (b) Container with built-in measure. (c) Tablet as used for treating bed nets to protect from mosquitoes transmitting malaria. (*Continued.*)

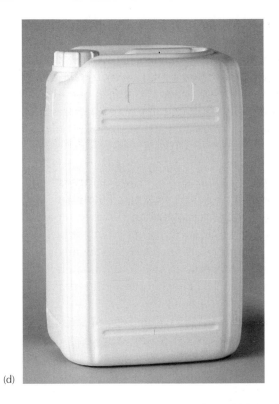

(d)

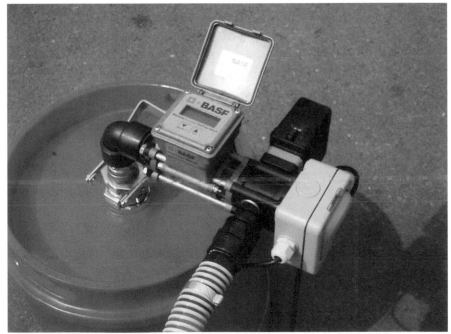

(e)

Fig 2.2   (*Continued.*) (d) Widely used plastic container. (e) Drum for closed-transfer system.

Retrospective assessment

Perhaps the most famous correlation of ill health and human activity was the link between lung cancer and the smoking of tobacco. An epidemiological study revealed that people exposed to the constituents of tobacco smoke, including nicotine, were undoubtedly more likely to suffer from lung cancer. Such epidemiological studies are more complex with pesticides, since the route and period of exposure to different pesticides is quite variable compared to direct inhalation of tobacco smoke by individuals. It has been suggested that people are exposed to pesticides through ingesting residues in food (see Chapter 7), through inhaling air contaminated by spray, or by direct dermal exposure when using pesticides. However, apart from those working in pesticide manufacturing facilities and users of pesticides, the quantities in each case are extremely low and mixed with many other chemicals. Air, especially in towns and cities, is also contaminated with vehicle exhausts, while many foods naturally contain many different chemicals.

Nevertheless, epidemiologists do study disease patterns to establish whether there are causal factors. One type of study is a cohort design, in which a group of people share a common characteristic. A study might include a group of certified spray applicators. At the start of the study, participants should initially be free of the disease under investigation, but their subsequent exposure to pesticides and health patterns are followed. The frequency of disease incidence between exposed and unexposed populations is then analysed to assess whether the exposure was the cause of ill health. If the group had been exposed at some time in the past, then a retrospective cohort study is carried out, based on the records of individuals and other relevant data, such as air-monitoring data. Cohort studies require the participation of a large number of people over a long period and are therefore expensive to conduct.

Where a study investigates, for example, the occurrence of a birth defect in a group of children, a case-control design can be used. Exposure data are sought from existing records or detailed questionnaires completed by the subjects, or next-of-kin, to compare the frequency of exposure with a similar unexposed control group, adjusted to allow for other factors that might have influenced the disease. Calculation of the ratio of disease incidence among those who were exposed or non-exposed with a similar group without the defect, who were exposed or not, can give an indication of whether the rate of defect incidence was higher, or not. Recall of details of exposure may not always be reliable if those suffering from a defect or disease are motivated to participate in the study.

Research by medical doctors and epidemiologists outside the laboratory is important as it can provide information that cannot be predicted from tests on non-human species. Information from multiple exposures under real-world conditions to a much larger population is crucial in confirming the verdicts from regulatory authorities. Nevertheless, care is needed in interpreting epidemiological studies unless the study has sound exposure data. Unfortunately, when news media report such studies, some aspects are overemphasised, without any scientific disclaimers given by the original authors, leading to sensational comments and scaremongering.

In Canada, an attempt was made to draw together information from selected published reports of epidemiological studies related to a number of human diseases and alleged pesticide exposure. The report (Sanborn *et al.*, 2004) acknowledged that epidemiology studies are difficult to interpret because of biases and confounding factors, making it difficult to establish any link between pesticide exposures and illnesses. This is especially important as people will also encounter other chemical and physical environmental effects that may have been responsible for the illness. A weakness of many studies is the use of surrogate information (sales data, crops grown, recall of what was applied) in the absence of being able to quantify what levels of pesticides the individuals were actually exposed to, and when these exposures occurred. Thus, in the absence of actual exposure data, it is not possible to assess whether pesticides could be the cause, and the general observation that exposure to pesticides should be curtailed as much as possible, especially for children, is undoubtedly correct. However, it is extremely difficult to unravel the causes of possible chronic effects, especially as recall of exposure events is very difficult and often vague.

In the UK, the Medical and Toxicological Panel of the Advisory Committee on Pesticides scrutinises, on an annual basis, the published papers on pesticides and human health to assess whether any regulatory action is required.

Environmental aspects

Potentially, there is a risk of pesticides adversely affecting all non-target organisms. Much depends on the toxicity of the pesticide, the application rate, and how it persists in the environment. Initially, the fate and behaviour of the pesticide are assessed with calculations of the predicted environmental concentration (PEC). In the USA, the PEC is referred to as an estimated environmental concentration (EEC). These environmental concentrations are calculated for soil, water, sediment and air. As it would be extremely expensive to measure the concentration of pesticide in many different situations, models are used to predict the PEC based on the physical properties of the chemical, and validated in certain situations by actual measurements. An example of PEC_{water} (Table 2.2) shows the decrease with distance and over time.

Table 2.2   Predicted environmental concentration (PEC) values (µg/l) in water for a pesticide

	Days after treatment		
Distance to water (m)	0	7	14
0	530	450	390
5	50	45	40
10	25	20	15
50	1	0.9	0.8

Table 2.3   Three levels of tests on non-target organisms

Species	Tier 1 Acute toxicity	Tier 2 Reproduction test	Tier 3 Field test
Avian (e.g. bobwhite quail)	LD_{50}		
Freshwater fish (e.g. rainbow trout or minnows)	Fish LC_{50}	Effects on spawning	Fish life cycle study
Aquatic invertebrate (e.g. *Daphnia*, shrimp)	Invertebrate EC_{50}	Full life cycle	Simulated field test
Non-target invertebrates (e.g. honey bee and earthworms)	Acute LD_{50}	Effect of residues on foliage	Field test for pollination
Terrestrial plants (e.g. various crops)	Seed germination		
Aquatic plants (e.g. algae)	Plant vigour		

Table 2.4   Comparison of toxicity exposure ratio (TER) for two insecticides to fish when using two application rates

	Recommended dose		Reduced dose	
Pesticide	A	B	A	B
PEC_{water} (mg/l)	0.08	0.08	0.045	0.045
Fish acute toxicity				
LC (mg/l)	8.5	0.05	8.5	0.05
TER	106.25	0.625	188.9	1.1
Fish chronic NOEC				
mg/l	0.4	0.015	0.4	0.015
TER	5.0	0.17	8.88	0.33

In the approval system, data on the effect of key non-target species are required to make comparisons with the PEC. The toxicity exposure ratio (TER) is used to determine whether the risk to the organism is acceptable, or not. The TER is calculated from the LC_{50} or equivalent measure of the susceptibility of an organism divided by the PEC relevant to the situation in which the organism is living. Thus, the PEC_{water} is used to assess the TER for fish. A TER of <100 for acute risk to fish indicates a need for detailed higher tier risk assessment. For chronic risk, the TER is <10. In the USA, the calculated risk quotient is the inverse of TER – that is, the PEC is divided by the indicated toxic dose. The assessment of acute toxicity to different non-target organisms is confined to selected surrogate organisms (Table 2.3). These tests are followed by more specific tests relevant to the life cycle of the organism and the way in which the pesticide will be applied. For example, aldicarb is an extremely toxic insecticide and nematicide that has been used effectively in many countries, but will be phased out in the EU by 2007. This insecticide was only used as a low-percentage granule for soil treatment, but there were still instances of bird mortality where granules remained on the soil surface. The final tier is a simulated or real field test.

If two different pesticides are compared (Table 2.4) using Tier 1 data and the risk is not acceptable (as shown by pesticide B), then further data are needed from Tiers 2 or 3 to see if there is any way the pesticide can be used to reduce its toxicity to fish. This may be by changes in formulation, reduced dosage (if still effective against the pests), or a wider buffer zone to protect the water. Recognising that pesticide B is acutely toxic to fish (Table 2.4), the TER for acute toxicity at a reduced application rate and is changed with a lower PEC_{water} value. However, in this example it is still not acceptable, so further evaluation would be needed at Tier 2, especially as the chronic toxicity TER is unacceptable.

Similar data are generated for all the non-target organisms evaluated. The PEC_{soil} can vary with different crops, depending on the application rate, the frequency of application and the persistence of deposits in the soil. As the sensitivity of soil inhabitants can also vary, for example between species of earthworms, the TER needs to be calculated to relate to the particular circumstances where the pesticide will be used.

Changes in evaluating pesticides in relation to non-target arthropods have been proposed. These include the European Standard Characteristics of Non-Target Arthropod Regulatory Testing (ESCORT 2), which considers both in-field and off-field effects for spray treatments. This is likely to be most important for certain pesticides, such as insect growth regulators.

Companies developing new molecules assess their future prospects by carrying out a comprehensive risk assessment to ensure that their investment will lead to a commercially registered product. One example of a risk assessment for a novel insecticide spinosad was reported by Cleveland *et al.* (2001).

Endocrine disrupters

Some organisations concerned about safety have called for banning of certain pesticides, which are referred to as 'endocrine disrupters', or 'environmental estrogens'. The argument is that such chemicals could adversely affect hormone balance, or disrupt their action regulating the normal function of organs. In the media, claims of an epidemiological study that sperm counts of humans had declined by almost 50% over the past fifty years due to exposure to synthetic chemicals hit the headlines. Immediately, pesticides were implicated, despite our exposure to a whole range of different chemicals in the environment.

The EPA defines endocrine disrupters as chemicals, from both natural and man-made sources, which interfere with the synthesis, secretion, transport, binding action or elimination of natural hormones in the body. As with other chemicals, any effect depends on when and how large is the dose present in the body. Below a threshold dose, there will be no effect, and at very small doses above the threshold there may even be a beneficial effect. It is only at large doses that adverse effects would occur.

Many endocrine disruptors are thought to mimic hormones as their chemical properties are similar to hormones, and this allows them to bind to hormone-specific receptors on the cells of target organs. Like other chemical groups, endocrine disruptor chemistry and potency varies. The generally low potency of most endocrine disruptors means that a higher dose is required to obtain the same response as the hormone that they mimic.

No standard tests are available to establish whether a chemical is an endocrine disruptor, although assays of a large number of chemicals for endocrine disruptive activity are being undertaken in the USA by their Endocrine Disrupter Screening Programme (EDSP). Data from multi-generation animal studies would provide strong evidence if a pesticide had the potential to act as an endocrine disruptor, especially as any effects on reproduction are assessed.

Colborn *et al.* (1993) reported concerns about effects of these chemicals on humans and wildlife, but the procedures being used for risk assessment are not considered to be sustainable in the future (Bridges and Bridges, 2004). Among the pesticides that are claimed by organisations, such as Friends of the Earth, to have reproductive- and endocrine-disrupting effects are the herbicides 2,4-D, 2,4,5-T, alachlor, amitrole, atrazine, metribuzin, nitrofen and trifluralin. Some fungicides benomyl, mancozeb maneb, tributyltin, zineb and ziram, are also implicated, while the insecticides include aldicarb, carbaryl, chlordane, dicofol, dieldrin, DDT, endosulfan, heptachlor, lindane, methomyl, methoxychlor, parathion, synthetic pyrethroids and toxaphene.

This list has many different types of pesticides with a wide range of properties, toxicity and persistence. Where specific studies have been made, for example, with alligators and birds as well as rats, the effects on reproduction have been achieved only at very high doses. This has led to speculation by some toxicologists that exposure to lower doses of some chemicals in the environment could be unacceptable, but this does not take into account the normal excretion and breakdown that occur.

Approval in relation to efficacy

Manufacturers of new pesticides have to demonstrate that when the product is used as recommended it is effective against the pests for which it will be marketed. The aim is to stop application of an ineffective pesticide and to avoid unnecessary addition of another chemical into the environment. Data are required to support the label claims, especially the recommended dose, to show that the pesticide does not cause any damage to the crop or adversely affect yields, and that it is not so persistent that it could cause damage to a subsequent crop. New pesticides require a high level of activity against the pests in a series of trials on crops on which the pesticide is intended to be used. It has been argued that within an integrated pest management programme, there may be a need for certain products which may be less active against a pest, but nevertheless contribute to the overall control strategy, for example by not adversely affecting biological control agents.

As part of this data package, consideration is now required on a resistance management policy, should the pest become resistant to the pesticide or a chemical with a similar mode of action. Often, this requires the label to state the maximum number of applications or maximum amount of active ingredient applied per season in conjunction with similar or complementary products. Industry has established specialist groups to assess the occurrence of resistance in insects, fungi, weeds and rodents, and to develop strategies to offset this problem, so that appropriate information is available both within the agrochemical industry and to growers. A key concern of industry is that growers do not use less than the label-recommended rate. They consider that the label rate is established from the results of many trials and represents a robust rate that will be effective under a wide range of conditions. The label rate with Good Agricultural Practice (GAP) is set to satisfy retail outlets that produce should not exceed a maximum residue level (MRL). In some countries the user is bound to apply the label rate, but in some circumstances it will be too high and if a farmer applies a pesticide accurately at the right time, a lower than label dose will be effective. There is no evidence that using a low dose rate will increase the incidence of resistance to a pesticide, whereas using too high a dose is more likely to select a resistant pest population. Furthermore, reduced rates of pesticides fit IPM better, provided that natural enemy survival is sufficient to regulate the survivors of a chemical treatment.

Operator proficiency

In the UK, there are an estimated 60,500 spray operators using an estimated 53,000 sprayers on farms (Garthwaite, 2004). Spray operators may only apply a pesticide in the UK if they have received training and have passed a practical test arranged by the National Proficiency Test Council (NPTC). This is mandatory for all those involved in spraying who were born after 31st December 1964, and those who pass the test may join a National Register of Spray Operators (NRoSo). It is rather like a driving test, and ensures that users are fully aware of what they must do according to the label and understand how to calibrate their equipment. It was thought that fully trained operators would ensure their equipment was fully operational, but as with motor vehicles, the operator test is not sufficient. Following the mandatory equipment test introduced in other European countries, for example in Belgium (Braekman and Sonck, 2004), the Agricultural Engineers Association has set up a National Sprayer Testing Scheme (NSTS) in the UK. Continued training is needed as new developments take place.

Waste management

Under legislation in Europe, there are strict rules concerning the disposal of used pesticide containers when they are empty. Previously, small plastic containers, after they had been triple-rinsed, could be incinerated on the farm, but these must now be returned to authorised waste disposal companies. In some countries (e.g. France and Brazil), systems of collecting used containers have been introduced, while some manufacturers are supporting the use of multi-trip containers. The use of the latter with closed transfer systems (Fig. 2.2e and Fig. 4.6) is referred to also in Chapter 3. These problems are greater in remote tropical countries, where containers have a value for other purposes. For example, 200-litre drums are still the most economical method of long-range transport, but local repackaging is needed to ensure that small-scale farmers have their pesticides in appropriate quantities for use on small areas. Sachets of water-soluble pesticides, wrapped to prevent water access until used and containing sufficient for one knapsack sprayer, are ideal, but they tend to be expensive and are not suitable for all active ingredients and formulations. Sachets that are not water-soluble are now used in some areas and avoid the wastage that can occur once larger packaging has been opened. The safe disposal of empty sachets must be done with great care. Some products can be formulated as tablets, while for others small pack designs are being introduced.

This chapter has indicated that the approval of pesticides is only possible in the UK after a vast amount of information has been examined in detail to ensure that the pesticide's use does not incur an unacceptable risk to humans and the environment. In contrast to many countries, many pesticides are not approved as they are considered too toxic or too persistent and liable to build up in food chains. The certification of spray operators and examination of sprayers is designed to ensure that pesticides are applied as safely and judiciously as possible.

References

Anon (2000) *A Guide to Pesticide Regulation in the UK and the Role of the Advisory Committee on Pesticides (ACP)*. DEFRA.

Braekman, P. and Sonck, B. (2004) Accreditation according to EN 4504 as a guarantee for a correct, reliable and objective mandatory inspection of sprayers in Flanders, Belgium. *Aspects of Applied Biology* **71**, 35–40.

Bridges, J.W. and Bridges, O. (2004) Integrated risk assessment and endocrine disrupters. *Toxicology* **205**, 11–15.

Cleveland, C.B., Mayes, M.A. and Cryer, S.A. (2001) An ecological risk assessment for spinosad use on cotton. *Pest Management Science* **58**, 70–84.

Colborn, T, vom Saal, F.S. and Soto, A.M. (1993) Developmental effects of endocrine-disrupting chemicals in wildlife and humans. *Environmental Health Perspectives* **101**, 378–384.

Garthwaite, D.G. (2004) Summary of the results of a survey of current farm sprayer practices in the United Kingdom. *Aspects of Applied Biology* **71**, 19–26.

Hamilton, D., Ambrus, A., Dieterie, R., Felsot, A., Harris, C., Petersen, B., Racke, K., Wong, S.-S., Gonzalez, R., Tanaka, K., Earl, M., Roberts, G. and Bhula, R. (2004) Pesticide residues in food – acute dietary exposure. *Pest Management Science* **60**, 311–339.

Ngowi, A.V.F., Maeda, D.N., Wesseling, C., Partenen, T.J. Sanga, M.P. and Mbise, G. (2001) Pesticide-handling practices in agriculture in Tanzania: Observational data from 27 coffee and cotton farms. *International Journal of Occupational and Environmental Health* **7**, 326–332.

Renwick, A.G., Dome, J.L. and Walton, K. (2000) An analysis of the need for an additional uncertainty factor for infants and children. *Regulatory Toxicology and Pharmacology* **31**, 286–296.

Ross, J.H., Driver, J.H., Cochran, R.C., Thongsinthusak, T. and Krieger, R.I. (2001) Could pesticide toxicology studies be more relevant to occupational risk assessment? *Annals of Occupational Hygiene* **45** (Suppl. 1), S5–S17.

Sanborn, M., Cole, D., Kerr, K., Vakil, C., Sanin, L.H. and Bassil, K. (2004) *Pesticides Literature Review*. Ontario College of Family Physicians.

Solecki, R., Davies, L., Dellarco, V., Dewhurst, I., van Raaij, M. and Tritscher, A. (2005). Guidance on setting of acute reference dose (ARfD) for pesticides. *Food and Chemical Toxicology*, **43**, 1569–1593.

Woods, H.F. (Chairman) (2004) *Risk Assessment of Mixtures of Pesticides and Similar Substances*. Committee of Toxicity of Chemicals in Food, Consumer Products and the Environment Department of Health, London.

3 Application of pesticides

Pesticides are used in a wide range of environments. In most cases, the active ingredient is formulated so that it can be diluted with water and applied by forcing the liquid through a very small opening in a nozzle to form a spray that is targeted at the intended surfaces. From the nozzle the spray is subject to various factors, and only a proportion of the pesticide applied reaches its intended target (Fig. 3.1). Spraying equipment was first developed in France during the late nineteenth century, when farmers began to spray Bordeaux mixture (a copper fungicide) onto their vines (Lodeman, 1896). Initially, a hand-operated pump was used as part of a small tank carried on the user's back; the first knapsack sprayer. Soon, larger horse-drawn versions were designed, which were the forerunners of the tractor-operated equipment used by farmers today.

Apart from pesticide use on farms, these products are also used in homes through pressure-packs (often called aerosol cans) and in gardens with compression or knapsack sprayers. In the tropics, houses may be sprayed with insecticide to control mosquitoes and other disease vectors, although the impregnation of fibres used in the fabric of bed-nets is a recent development to minimise the transmission of malaria. Vector control also involves treatment of the mosquito breeding sites, such as water pools and ditches, with an insecticide aimed at killing the larvae, and by space treatments with vehicle-mounted or aerial equipment.

This chapter briefly describes the main types of pesticide application equipment in order to place the information in the following chapters into context.

Hydraulic sprayers

World-wide, most pesticides are applied through hydraulic sprayers of various size and complexity (Figs. 3.2–3.5). From the smallest knapsack to aerial equipment, the main parts are a tank, a pump and a set of nozzles, interconnected by pipes/hoses and control valves. More detailed information is provided in other books on different types of sprayers (Matthews, 2000) and their use on different crops that are treated with pesticides (Matthews, 1999).

The spray produced will depend on the design of the nozzle, its shape and size, as well as the pressure at which it is operated. Traditionally, the

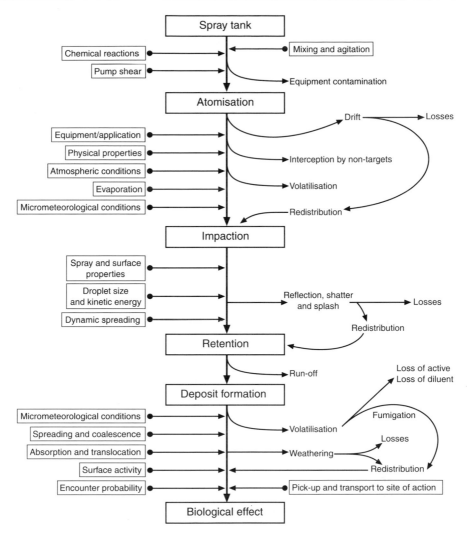

Fig. 3.1 The dose transfer process, showing the complexity of effects on movement of the pesticide from the sprayer to achieve a biological effect (reproduced from Matthews, 2000).

pesticide was diluted in a large volume of water, and often 1000 litres or more were applied per hectare to crops. Once the exposed foliage was wetted, much of the liquid dripped to the ground and was wasted. This technique is still used in some parts of the world, but – with farm size increasing and a shrinking labour force – the need to enhance field work rates, the cost of collecting and transporting sufficient water to fields, and the increasing recognition of the wastage of chemicals with high-volume spraying has led to the application of much lower spray volumes. In the UK, the recent trend has been to reduce sprays on large-scale farms from over 200 litres per hectare to between 80 and 150 litres per hectare. At the same time, the

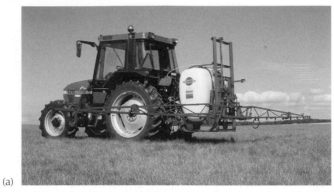

(a)

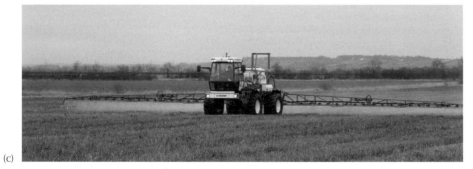

(b)

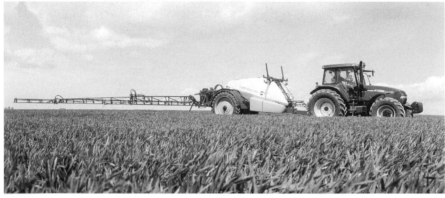

(c)

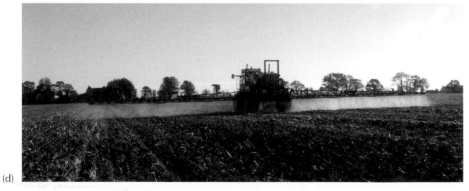

(d)

Fig. 3.2 Tractor sprayer: (a) Mounted on 3-point linkage; (b) trailed; (c, d) self-propelled with part (d) showing wide boom (24 m). (*Continued*.)

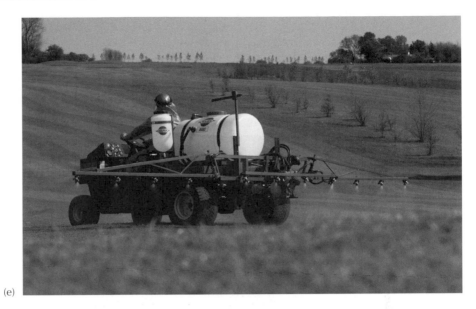

(e)

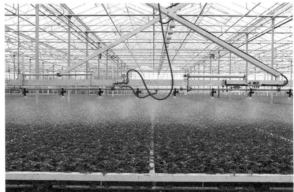

(f)

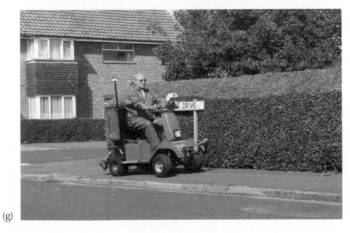

(g)

Fig. 3.2   (*Continued.*) (e) Turf sprayer; (f) boom sprayer in glasshouse; (g) local authority sprayer. (Photographs (a), (b) and (e) from Hardi International; (c) and (d) from Househam Sprayers; (f) from GAM; (g) from Nomix.)

speed of travel across fields is increasing. Boom widths have increased, with 18–24-m booms being preferred to increase work rates, and even wider booms (e.g. 36 m) where the land is very flat. The choice of boom width is usually dictated as a multiple of the seeder width; thus, with a 4-m seeder a 20-m boom would be selected to accommodate the 'tramlines' that allow tractor access at all stages of crop growth.

Apart from the tractor-mounted, trailed or self-propelled boom sprayers used in arable farming, there are downwardly directed air-assisted sprayers for treating field crops (Fig. 3.3), but air-assisted sprayers have been developed primarily for treating orchards (Fig. 3.4). Various designs are used with axial, centrifugal and cross-flow fans to move air with droplets into crop canopies. Interest in air-assisted sprayers for treating arable crops has increased where it is important to reduce spray drift. However, the foliage has to filter the droplets projected into the canopy, otherwise there may be more drift if the air bounces back from the ground.

Hydraulic nozzles

Typically, nozzles have been designed to provide either a cone or flat, fan-shaped sheet of spray (Fig. 3.6). The latter has always been preferred on large tractor equipment, where the nozzles are mounted across a horizontal boom. Cone nozzles in contrast have been used on hand-operated

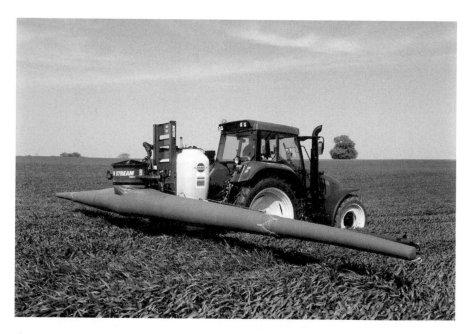

Fig. 3.3 Air-assisted boom sprayer provides a downwardly directed flow of air into the crop canopy.

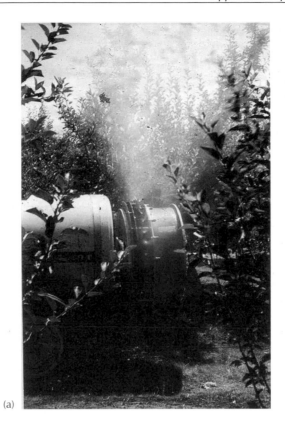

(a)

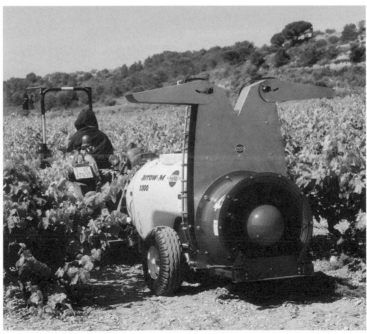

(b)

Fig. 3.4 Air-assisted sprayers for bush and tree crops. (a) Axial fan sprayer in apples; (b) in vines.

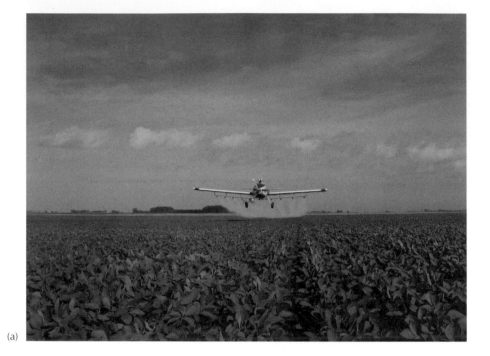

(a)

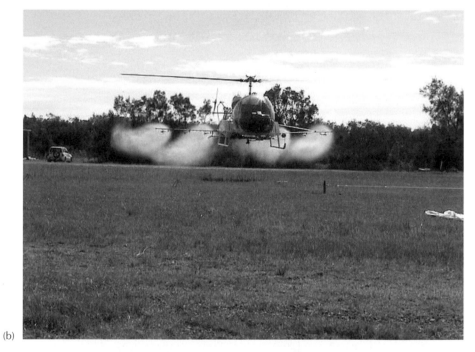

(b)

Fig. 3.5   (a) Aerial sprayer; (b) helicopter spraying. (*Continued.*)

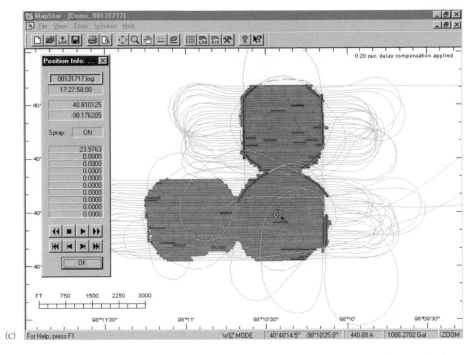

Fig. 3.5 (*Continued.*) (c) GPS tracking allows more accurate treatment and recording exactly where spray was applied from aircraft.

sprayers and for equipment used in orchards in which spray droplets are projected into the crop by a blast of air from a fan. The use of air-assistance has increased in arable crops, by using air that is ducted through a sleeve to create an air-curtain that propels droplets downwards across the width of a spray boom. In this way, there is better penetration of crop canopies and spray droplets are less prone to downwind movement across the top of the crop canopy. Nozzles may be damaged where water supplies are poor, as the orifice in the soft metal can soon be eroded by particles of sand or other debris. To overcome this problem, some nozzles are made either in ceramic or stainless steel. The development of hard-wearing polymers has enabled farmers to use moulded plastic nozzles rather than the more traditional machined designs. The change in manufacturing technique provides nozzle tips of consistently high quality, but inevitably erosion of the orifice will occur. However, the nozzle tips are also more readily changed since they can be fitted (using a bayonet retaining cap) either individually at each mounting point or in matched sets across the boom to meet a range of contrasting application needs. Flat-fan nozzle tips are now colour-coded to an international standard so that farmers are able to select a set of the same output. The colour does not indicate the spray angle or type of tip. A filter, often of 50 mesh, is fitted into the nozzle body to prevent blockages of the

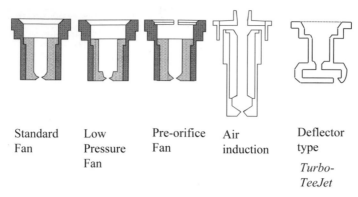

Standard Fan	Low Pressure Fan	Pre-orifice Fan	Air induction	Deflector type
				Turbo-TeeJet

Fig. 3.6 Types of hydraulic fan nozzles (reproduced from Matthews, 2000).

small orifice while spraying. A check valve is used at the nozzle to prevent liquid dripping from the lance or boom.

Farmers can spend large amounts of money on pesticides, and often forget that by investing in new nozzle tips they can save money. A farmer can spend £10–£50 per hectare for pesticide products, so if we assume £21 per hectare, including mixing an adjuvant, the total cost of chemical is £10,500 for 500 hectares. If the nozzle is eroded and the flow rate has increased by 5%, the farmer could spend £11,025 – an extra £525 – whereas the cost of new nozzle tips across the boom would be less than £75.

Until laser equipment was developed to measure the size of the spray droplets from different nozzles, the main criterion was the output of the nozzle and the shape of the spray pattern. However, detailed assessment of the spray spectra confirmed that hydraulic nozzles produce droplets of a very wide range of sizes: some extremely small droplets are less than 100 micrometres (μm) in diameter, while others exceed 500 μm. This range of droplet sizes varies with nozzle design and use and can – with some pesticides – have a major effect on efficacy, crop selectivity and losses from beyond the intended treatment area. Drift losses are not just recent issues. After some hot weather in the UK in May 1976, concern increased that herbicides, which were applied to cereals, were adversely affecting vegetable crops downwind of treated fields. Investigations revealed that apart from volatile spray deposits being carried downwind, there was a risk that the smallest spray droplets were also liable to be carried by air movement out of the treated fields. In consequence, the British Crop Protection Council's Working Group on Chemical Applications initiated a study of droplet spectra from different nozzles. This led to a Spray Classification Scheme (Fig. 3.7) in which different sprays could be classified as 'fine', 'medium' or 'coarse' (Doble *et al.*, 1985). Nozzles that produced a high proportion of droplets in a 'very fine' category were not recommended for treating fields, because of the hazard of drift, although they could be used in glasshouses or other indoor

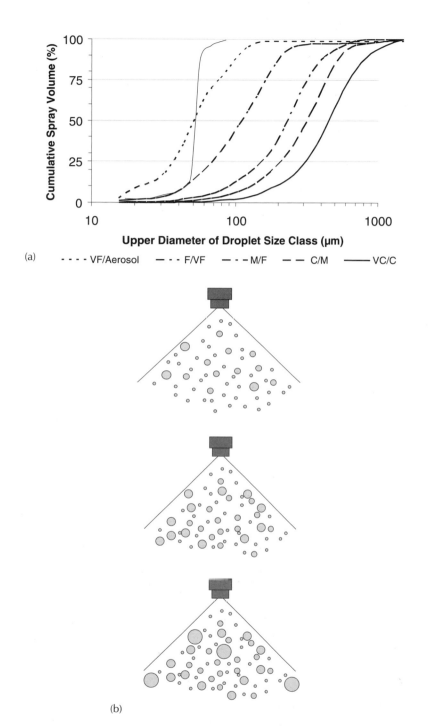

Fig. 3.7 (a) BCPC spray classification with hydraulic nozzles (IPARC). The more vertical line is for a rotary atomiser. The position of this line depends on atomiser speed and flow rate. (b) Diagram showing range of droplets sizes within a fine, medium and coarse spray.

situations, for which subsequent studies have separated 'mists' and 'fogs' within the 'very fine' category (Matthews and Bateman, 2004). At the other extreme, 'very coarse' sprays were generally not recommended as the large droplets tend to bounce off foliage, as leaves tend to have a waxy surface. This system of classification was modified to include a drift potential factor (Southcombe *et al.*, 1997) and to define more exactly the boundaries between the different categories. With further modifications this system of classification has been adopted in Europe and the USA. In the American standard, 'extra coarse' is an additional category. Nozzle manufacturers have included information on spray quality in their catalogues and other data are available on web sites such as www.dropdata.net.

Most farmers would use a 'medium' spray, but even with these nozzles some of the spray droplets can be carried downwind. This is discussed further in Chapters 5 and 6. However, in an effort to improve spraying, nozzles have been designed in which air is mixed with the spray liquid. In some cases air is forced into the nozzle using a compressor, while in others air is sucked into the nozzle using a Venturi. 'Twin-fluid' nozzles in which air is mixed with the spray liquid inside the nozzle have been developed to cope with different tractor speeds (from 6 to 20 km/h) and thus different flow rates, while maintaining a similar droplet size range (Combellack and Miller, 1999). Spray quality can be adjusted in the tractor cab without changing nozzles. This allows a very coarse spray to be applied adjacent to sensitive areas, such as a water-course, and then change quickly to a medium or fine spray to optimise spray deposition over the remainder of the field

Nozzles which suck in the air, known as air induction (AI) nozzles (Nozzle to right of Fig. 3.6) have become popular in Europe and elsewhere. Several different manufacturers have produced AI nozzles with different coarse spray spectra (Piggott and Matthews, 1999). To understand differences between these nozzles, Butler Ellis *et al.* (2002) investigated design parameters. Increasing both the Venturi throat diameter and final orifice size increased airflow rate but, compared to the final orifice size, air intake did not markedly affect droplet size. However, the proportion of very small droplets from AI fan nozzles is significantly less than with standard fan nozzles (Fig. 3.8), so the risk of downwind drift is reduced. With air entrapped inside them, the larger droplets are then less likely to bounce off foliage; the large – but slower – droplet is 'cushioned' at impact. However, the efficacy of some herbicides has been eroded by the more extensive use of low-pressure nozzles producing larger drop sizes, especially where the target surface is a vertical stem (e.g. grass weed). To overcome this problem, nozzles can be angled to project spray more directly at the target surface.

Field experiments have shown that variations in boom height, nozzle size, forward speed and nozzle operating pressure all affect the potential drift. The scale of drift risk is further compounded by the characteristics of the surface over which drift is measured, as surface friction and meteorological

Spray with droplets <100µm

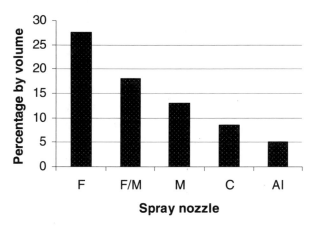

Fig. 3.8 Percentage by volume of droplets smaller than 100 µm, showing least spray in small droplets with air-induction nozzles.

variables all influence the movement of droplets while airborne (Bache and Johnstone, 1992). Thus, variation between individual trials/replicates makes model verification difficult (Holterman *et al.*, 1997), but does supply some comparative data to provide better recommendations on nozzle selection in relation to drift. Some models have under-predicted spray drift (Phillips and Miller, 1999), while other studies have shown that the position of nozzles on the boom and their spacing also influence drift potential (Murphy *et al.*, 2000).

While air-induction nozzles reduce drift, coverage is not so good on certain targets such as grass weeds (e.g. black grass seedlings prior to the three-leaf stage) (Powell *et al.*, 2003). Adaptations by angling an air-induction nozzle have subsequently been developed, for example to improve efficacy of late fungicide sprays on cereals (Robinson *et al.*, 2003). However, for improved coverage with small droplets, an external air-jet directed at the output of a fan nozzle causes improved break-up of the spray and entrains the small droplets within the air-stream, thus achieving less drift with a finer spray (Matthews and Thomas, 2000a; Matthews and Thomas, 2000b).

In row crops it is possible to spray a narrow band of pesticide either along the crop row or inter-row, depending on requirements. This is possible with 'even-spray' fan nozzles. The use of these has not been extensive, but may increase with genetically modified crops, which allow certain herbicides to be sprayed over the crop. Confining the pesticide to a narrow strip not only reduces the cost of treatment, but also allows the integration of other techniques such as inter-row hoeing.

International standards for hydraulic nozzles enable farmers to select the most appropriate nozzle for a particular pest problem. Colour coding of flat fan nozzles shows what their 'throughput' is at a specified pressure. All makes of nozzle should also fit the standard size nozzle body. Nozzle bodies do vary in terms of their fitting to the boom and type of retaining cap (bayonet or screw). Some booms have nozzle turrets so that different types of nozzle can be selected in the field. On advanced equipment, with modern control equipment in the tractor cab (Fig. 3.9), each nozzle has a solenoid valve to enable the nozzle to be computer-controlled, spraying sections of a field in relation to GIS/GPS data, for example when spraying patches of weeds rather than the whole field. The selection of a nozzle involves deciding the spray pattern (fan, cone), spray angle (e.g. 80°), output (litres/min) and spray quality at the desired operating pressure. The sprayer must also be calibrated to check the output is that required at the forward speed of the sprayer.

Sprayer testing

In several countries in Europe, it is now mandatory for a sprayer to be checked at regular intervals to ensure that farmers' maintain their equipment to a minimum standard. The check is equivalent to the routine inspection of vehicles, required before a vehicle can be taxed. In the UK, the National Sprayer Testing Scheme, operated by the Agricultural Engineers Association

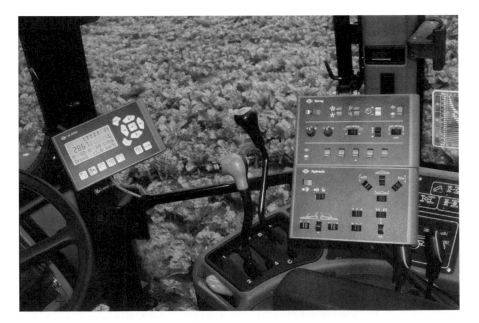

Fig. 3.9   Modern control equipment in tractor cab (photograph Hardi International).

(AEA) has been voluntary, but under the Voluntary Initiative, farmers were encouraged to submit their tractor sprayers to test centres. However, many feel it should be made compulsory. Among the first 8000 sprayers tested in the UK, 50% needed remedial treatment to pass the assessment. Faults were due to leakages (33%), poor hosing (15%), worn/inaccurate nozzles (20%) and inaccurate pressure gauges (14%).

Rotary atomisers

A major criticism of hydraulic nozzles is the wide range of sizes that are produced. A narrower droplet spectrum can be achieved by using a rotary atomiser or spinning disc. With these, the average droplet size is dependent upon the speed at which the outer surface of the rotating nozzle travels. Higher speeds produce smaller droplets. Initially, these were largely confined to laboratory studies, but where ultra-low volumes (ULV) (<5 litres per hectare) and very low volumes (VLV) are applied the rotary atomiser is usually better as the orifice in the flow constrictor is less likely to block. Equipment with rotary atomisers/spinning discs have been used mainly in arid areas, such as cotton-growing areas in Africa (Fig. 3.10a) and for locust control, and on aircraft (see Fig. 3.5). With slow rotational speeds, usually around 2000 rpm, small hand-carried spinning-disc sprayers have also been used for herbicide treatments in amenity areas and in forests, as droplets are consistently large enough to minimise spray drift (Fig. 3.10b).

Compression sprayers

These are popular for garden use. Most have a small plastic tank (<10 litres) and a hand-operated pump also provides the lid (Fig. 3.11a). A small lance has usually been fitted with a trigger valve and an adjustable cone nozzle. Settings can vary from a straight jet to a wide cone, the latter having the finest spray while the pressure is high. Spray quality will vary depending on the pressure and the way the nozzle is adjusted. Apart from the extreme positions of the nozzle, seldom can it be used consistently at intermediate settings. Unfortunately, adjusting the nozzle requires touching the nozzle, thus exposing hands to pesticide, so it is not recommended for general use and should be replaced by a standard fan or cone nozzle. A compression sprayer tank is not completely filled, so there is an airspace pressurised by pumping. As spray is applied, the pressure in the tank decreases and so users have to stop after a while and re-pressurise the tank. Ideally, a control flow valve is fitted to ensure uniform pressure at the nozzle. These sprayers are also used for treating wall surfaces in dwellings and warehouses, for example by pest control operators (Fig. 3.11b).

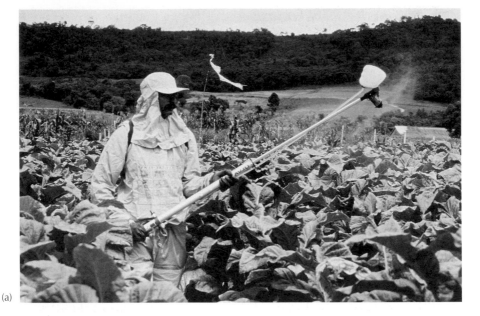

(a)

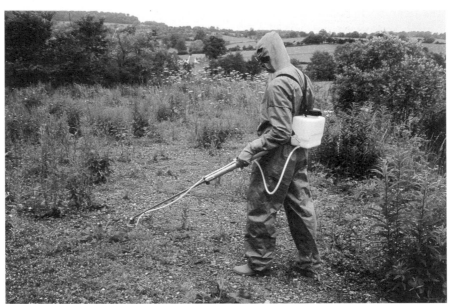

(b)

Fig. 3.10   Rotary atomiser CDA spinning disc sprayer. (a) Insecticide application on tobacco in Brazil; (b) applying herbicide (photographs Micron).

Knapsack sprayers

The lever-operated knapsack sprayer (Fig. 3.12a–c) requires continual pumping, in contrast to the compression sprayer, and is designed to pump the spray liquid, rather than air. It is probably the most widely used type

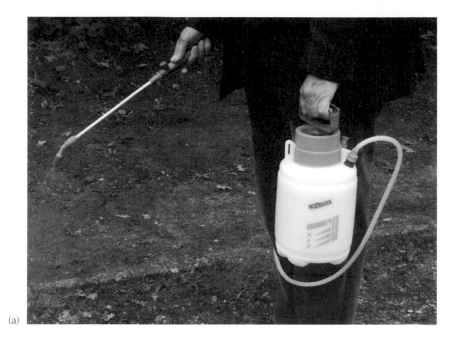

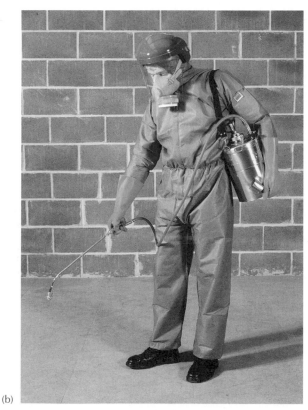

Fig. 3.11   (a) Small compression sprayer; (b) pest control operator with compression sprayer in a warehouse (photographs GAM and Kilgerm Group Ltd.).

of sprayer, being suitable for small farms and all areas inaccessible to vehicle equipment. The design of these sprayers has improved with modern manufacturing techniques and efforts to meet international standards, such as the minimum requirements for these sprayers published by FAO (Anon, 2000). The end of the lance should allow any type of hydraulic nozzle to be fitted so that the spray output and pattern meet the specific requirements for different pesticides and crops. Although the majority of these knapsack sprayers have a manually operated pump, some have a pump driven by an electric motor with a rechargeable battery. Some have a petrol-driven engine (usually two-stroke engine). Some engine-driven knapsack sprayers also have a fan to provide an air-stream to project the spray into trees and other crops. These are referred to as knapsack mistblowers (Fig. 3.12d), and are fitted with an air-shear nozzle or, in some cases, a rotary atomiser. Knapsack mistblowers tend to apply lower volumes and thus use sprays with a higher concentration of pesticide.

Home and garden use

Traditionally, some pesticides – especially insecticides – are sold as low-concentration dusts in 'puffer' packs. This allows small areas, such as around doorways and under sinks where cockroaches or ants occur, to be treated. The amount of dust emitted from individual puffs can vary depending on the amount in the container, the angle at which it is used, and the severity

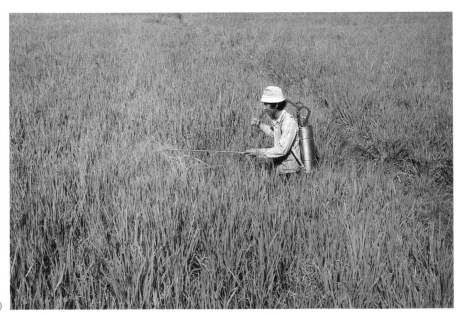

(a)

Fig. 3.12 (a) Lever-operated knapsack sprayer used in rice. (*Continued.*)

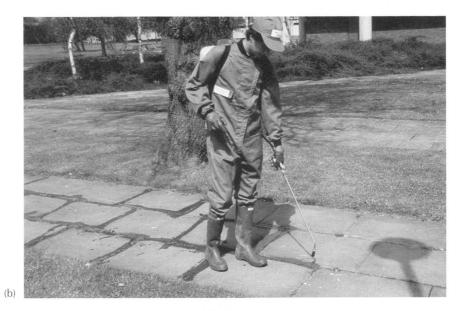

(b)

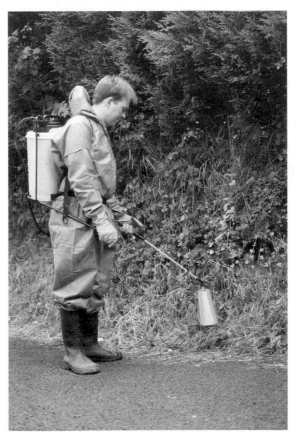

(c)

Fig. 3.12 (*Continued.*) (b) Spraying pavement to control weeds; (c) with shield around nozzle to protect spray from wind. (*Continued.*)

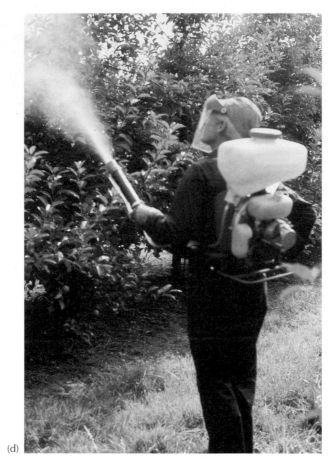

(d)

Fig. 3.12   *(Continued.)* (d) Knapsack mistblower.

of squeezing the container. In many situations the application of 'gels' or other techniques of pest management have replaced dusts.

Pressure packs, often referred to as aerosol cans, are a very popular means of spraying small quantities of pesticide. The chemical is dissolved in a solvent and sealed in a robust container with a propellant (compressed or liquefied gas). Fluorinated hydrocarbons are no longer used as propellant, and have largely been replaced by compressed air or butane. Operating the valve in the top of the can allows the pressure within the can to force liquid up a dip-tube and through the valve, which is also designed as a nozzle. Propellant reaching the atmosphere causes the liquid pesticide to break up into droplets. Depending on the volatility of the solvent and other factors, the droplet size produced can vary, but for insecticide application it tends to be less than 30 µm.

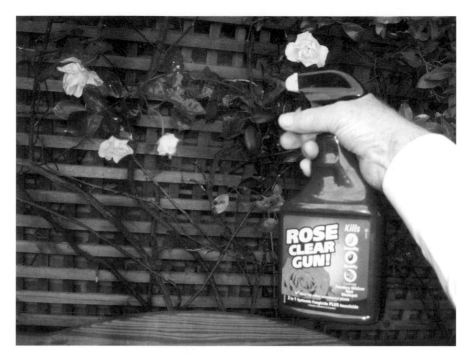

Fig. 3.13   Garden sprayer (photograph GAM).

A less expensive method of producing an aerosol with a hand-operated pump is to use a Flit gun. The small container can be refilled with pesticide. A small air pump, similar to a bicycle pump, is used to create a jet of air across the top of a dip tube to atomise the liquid and propel the droplets into the atmosphere.

Pre-diluted pesticides may also be sold in plastic containers with a trigger-operated cone nozzle (Fig. 3.13). These sprayers are very useful, where only small area, such as a few rose bushes, need treatment.

Weed wipers

When there is a risk of spray drift even over a very short distance to a sensitive plant, it has been possible to apply a translocated broad-spectrum herbicide, such as glyphosate with an absorbent sponge-like material, the 'wick' which is attached to a reservoir of the herbicide (Fig. 3.14). Weed wipers need to be designed so that the wick is sufficiently wet to transfer chemical to the weed, but not so wet that the herbicide drips from it. By touching surfaces, the wick can become dirty and affect chemical transfer. Equipment can be mounted on a tractor, or be hand-carried. They have been used to control specific weeds in set-aside and managed buffer zones.

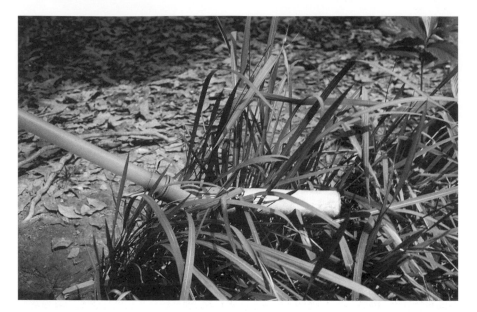

Fig. 3.14   Weed wiper (photograph GAM).

Space treatment equipment

Specialised equipment is used to apply small droplets inside warehouses, glasshouses and other spaces where flying insects need to be controlled (Fig. 3.15). The same equipment is occasionally used for applying certain fungicides, and also for treating outdoor areas where adult mosquitoes and other disease vectors require control. Small droplets are used so that they remain suspended in air as long as possible, although in still air even the smallest droplets will gradually fall by gravity over several hours on to exposed horizontal surfaces.

The use of thermal foggers was the main method of producing droplets smaller than 25 μm by vaporising the liquid containing the insecticide at about 400–500°C and allowing the vapour to condense as a dense white cloud of very small droplets. The insecticide was normally mixed with odourless kerosene or equivalent, but the trend is towards water-miscible products, that have to be mixed with a 'carrier'. Small hand-carried thermal foggers generally have a pulse-jet engine. Rather than use a high temperature, cold foggers use a vortex of air to shatter the spray into small droplets. Most vehicle-mounted cold foggers have a 16–20 hp engine, to drive a blower that provides low-pressure air to a vortical nozzle. Other cold fog equipment, which is electrically operated, can be set up with a timer to treat a space, such as a glasshouse, when not occupied. In contrast, thermal fogging equipment must not be left unattended due to fire risk. Insecticides formulated for cold fogs are increasingly diluted in water, but some incorporate a chemical

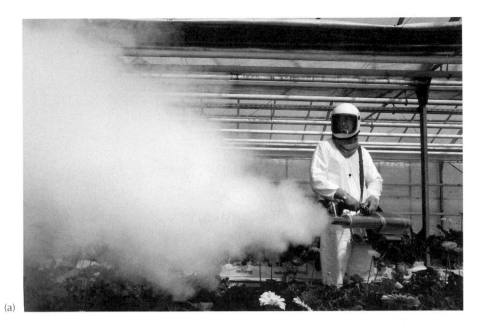

(a)

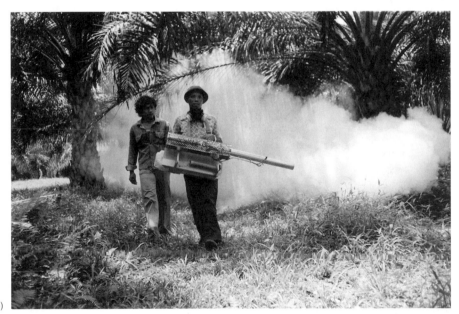

(b)

Fig. 3.15   Space treatments. (a) Thermal fogging in a glasshouse; (b) in a plantation. (*Continued.*)

which forms a film on the surface of droplets to reduce evaporation and thus prevent droplets shrinking and becoming too small.

Small droplets in glasshouses will be sucked out through gaps in the structure due to wind passing over the structure. However, if the building is well constructed, a fog can remain effective for several hours, before vents

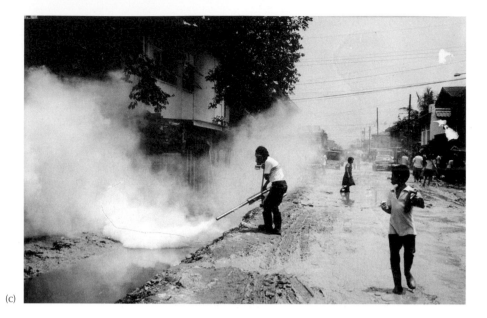

(c)

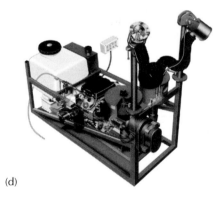

(d)

Fig. 3.15   (*Continued.*) (c) Vector control; (d) vehicle-mounted cold fogger. (*Continued.*)

are opened to ventilate the area and access is allowed. Respiratory protective equipment (RPE) must be worn when operating fogging equipment inside buildings, such as warehouses and glasshouses.

Granule application

A few pesticides are formulated as dry granules and used directly by incorporation into the soil to control pests, such as potato cyst nematode, or spread over the ground or crop to control slugs or weeds. Manually operated granule applicators have been used to apply nematicides on bananas. The nemati-

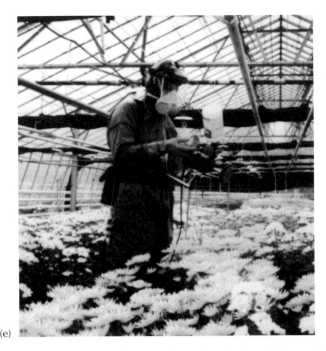

(e)

Fig 3.15   (*Continued.*) (e) Rotary nozzle mist application in a glasshouse (photograph Micron).

cides are often highly toxic pesticides that are considered too hazardous to apply as sprays. Granules are less easy to meter accurately compared with pumping a liquid through nozzles. Specialised equipment has been developed, which can also incorporate closed transfer of the product directly to the dispensing hopper. Care is needed to ensure the toxic pesticides are not left on the soil surface such that birds are exposed to the small particles.

Seed treatment

This is an important method of pesticide use, normally as a systemic fungicide or insecticide aimed at protecting the young seedlings, but sometimes with a safener to protect the seedlings from the effects of a herbicide. Seeds may be pelleted and also provided with some nutrients. Localised treatment reduces the dose applied. Prophylactic treatment is generally cost-effective where soil pathogens may drastically reduce seedling survival. Any early insect attack by sucking pests can also be controlled when a spray would be very inefficient due to the small size of the seedling relative to the ground area. Some seed may remain on the soil surface after drilling. De Snoo and Luttik (2004) estimated from field data that for risk assessment, the percentage of seed remaining on the soil surface was 3.3% for standard drilling in the spring, and 9.2% in the autumn, but this was reduced to 0.5% with precision drilling.

Storage of pesticides and equipment

It is essential that pesticides are stored safely as the concentrated formulations pose the most risk to human health and the environment. Equipment is best stored separately away from chemicals. In the UK, commercial pesticide stores must be inspected annually to ensure that the building is soundly constructed with fire-resistant materials, is well-lit and ventilated on a suitable site with adequate capacity and segregation of products. Pesticides must never be stored in places where flooding is possible, or where they might spill or leak into wells, drains, groundwater or surface water. Pesticide stores should be bunded and have a sump to prevent spillages reaching watercourses. This is also important if a fire occurs and water is used to quench the flames.

The building must be dry and frost-free, with appropriate warning signs and secure against theft and vandalism. Suitable access and exits must also be provided with provision to contain any spillage or leakages. Staff must be trained. The following guidelines also need to be followed where pesticides are stored on farms:

- Avoid excessive quantities in stock by having only the amount needed in the near future.
- Keep all pesticides in a locked, ideally separate store or cabinet in a well-ventilated utility area, barn or garden shed, and ensure that any spillages do not seep into the ground or enter watercourses. Where small quantities are involved, the locked cabinet must be high enough to be out of reach of children. Never store pesticides in the same area as food, animal feed or medical supplies. In some countries, where pesticides were in the same general stores, legislation now insists that pesticides are sold from separate shops.
- Pesticides must be stored in their original containers, with the label listing ingredients, directions for use, and first aid steps in case of accidental poisoning. Follow all storage instructions on the pesticide label. *Never* transfer pesticides to soft drink bottles or other containers. Children or others may mistake them for something to eat or drink.
- In domestic use, always use containers that are child-resistant and close the container tightly after using the product. However, 'child-resistant' does not mean 'child-proof', so extra care is needed to store the container properly in a locked cabinet as described above.
- If the contents of the container cannot be identified, or how old the contents are, follow advice on safe disposal.

- Further information on storage is available at http://www.hse.gov.
  uk/pubns/ais16.pdf; http://www.epa.gov/pesticides/regulating/
  store.htm; http://entweb.clemson.edu/pesticid/saftyed/storage.
  htm; http://www.environment-agency.gov.uk/netregs; http://www.
  agregister.co.uk

Timing and number of spray applications

In some crops, especially in the developing countries, recommendations
were simplified by recommending that sprays were repeated at weekly,
10-day or longer intervals on a regular calendar schedule. This meant that
some applications might be made when no pest or disease was present, so
the trend has been to recommend crop monitoring and only to apply a pesticide if the pest or disease economic threshold was exceeded. That is, if pest
numbers continue to increase, loss of crop yield and/or quality will reduce
the farmer's income unless appropriate control measure are undertaken.

Scouting

Crop monitoring can be done in various ways depending on the pest and
crop.

Some farmers employ specialist consultants to 'walk' their crops and
decide whether a pesticide is needed. In some crops, routine scouting is
essential to assess if an insect population needs control. Such scouting can
be assisted by using pheromone or various types of sticky trap to sample
the pest population. While traps may indicate the presence of a pest, the
scout may still need to examine the crop as trap catches may not be directly
correlated with the pest population within the crop. Where a disease such
as potato blight is anticipated, mini-meteorological stations close to the crop
can monitor temperature, humidity and rainfall so that the farmer can assess
with the assistance of Decision Support Systems, whether conditions will
favour the disease.

Some pre-emergence herbicides could be applied before weeds were
present, often at the time a crop was sown, but the trend has been to apply
selective herbicides when crop walking indicates that weeds are present in
sufficient numbers to justify treatment. With herbicide-tolerant, GM crops,
a broad-spectrum herbicide can be applied later in the season. Small cloches
can be used to accelerate germination or growth of latent weeds to aid identification and likely control measures.

Generally, economics dictate the minimum number of applications, but
some crops may require several different pesticides over a period of some
weeks. Typical programmes for selected crops are shown in Table 3.1. The
development of insect-resistant GM crops, such as Bt cotton, will reduce the

number of spray applications typically needed on the crop for a particular pest. Some pesticides are applied as late sprays to protect the harvested produce during storage.

The ideal situation is when a pesticide is accurately timed and the dose minimised to keep pest populations just below the economic threshold. Optimising an application of herbicide, as with other pesticides, depends on timeliness, as the dose required for weeds or insects increases with their size or age. Delaying a herbicide spray by a short period (e.g. from the three- to four-leaf stage) can increase the dose required by 50% or more (Miller, 2003).

This dose should be applied only where it is needed in the crop. However, targeting the dose to the particular biological site where action is needed is difficult, and in reality the farmer generally has to spray the whole field, although at least for weeds research has indicated that spraying individual patches of weeds is possible. In some situations, a lower dose of insecticide has the advantage that it will be less harmful to beneficial insects in integrated pest management. Angling nozzles has helped to increase deposits on vertical target such as wheat stems.

Table 3.1   Examples of spray programmes for: (a) winter wheat in southern England; (b) an orchard crop; and (c) cotton. (*Continued.*)

(a) Winter wheat. Specialist walks through crops to decide whether pest infestation justifies a treatment. Actual dates will vary with seasonal temperatures and other climatic factors

Growth stage	Reason for spraying	Possible treatment
3 leaf (late October)	blackgrass annual meadow grass broad-leaved weeds aphids - BYDV**	isoproturon* + diflufenican pyrethroid
GS30-31 (early April)	growth regulation, wild oats if required	chlormequat, fenoxaprop-P-ethyl + mineral oil
GS32 (late April)	*Septoria tritici* mildew if required poppies, charlock cleavers if required	tebuconazole chlorothalonil fenpropidin metsulfuron-methyl fluroxypyr
GS33 (early May)	growth regulation (weak straw cultivars)	2-chloroethylphosphonic acid + mepiquat chloride + non-ionic wetter
GS39 (late May)	*Septoria* mildew if required	epoxiconazole fenpropidin
GS59 (June)	ear diseases if required aphids if required	epoxiconazole pirimicarb

*Maximum dosage 2.5 ai/ha/year
**On barley a seed treatment with imidicloprid mixed with fungicides for loose smut control will also reduce aphid populations to check barley yellow dwarf virus.

Table 3.1   (*Continued.*) (b) Apple orchards. (Research is investigating a significant reduction in the number of sprays on apples. In some countries more insecticide sprays were applied for codling moth control, but alternative methods are being investigated.)

Growth stage	Pest/Disease	Pesticide	Comments
Bud burst	scab/canker	pyrifenox + dithianon	Ensure wetting of wood with HV spray Early scab control is very important
Mouse ear	rust mite canker scab/canker	pirimiphos methyl carbendazim pyrifenox + captan	If mite count is high where canker risk occurs
Late green cluster	lepidopteran pests, aphids, capsids, rust mite sawfly scab/mildew scab	chlorpyrifos sticky traps pyrifenox + captan	Inspect orchards Put in orchards low rate of captan to suppress scab
Pink bud	scab/mildew tortrix nutrition	pyrifenox fenoxycarb urea	Add captan to enhance scab protection High risk to bees
Blossom	scab/mildew	pyrifenox	Time sprays to start and end of blossom if possible
First flower	sawfly/canker	carbendazim	Some control of sawfly obtained with carbendazim
Petal fall	caterpillars, aphids, capsid	chlorpyrifos	Risk to bees Use pheromone traps for codling and tortrix moths
	sawfly aphids codling/ tortrix red spider mite scab nutrition	HCH pirimicarb fenoxycarb fenpyroximate pyrifenox	Apply sprays only if orchard at risk
+ 10 days	scab/mildew	pyrifenox + captan	Reduce rate if scab risk is low
+ 10 days	clouded drab moth canker scab/mildew	carbendazim pyrifenox + captan	Inspect orchards apply chlorpyrifos if necessary
+ 10 days	scab mildew nutrition	captan bupirimate calcium chloride	Only if necessary if high risk use
+ 10 days	summer fruit tortrix/ codling scab mildew nutrition	chlorpyrifos captan bupirimate calcium chloride	Spray 7–10 days after number of moths in pheromone traps exceeds threshold only if necessary

(*Continued.*)

Table 3.1   (b) (*Continued.*)

Growth stage	Pest/Disease	Pesticide	Comments
Early July	summer fruit tortrix/ codling	chlorpyrifos	Spray 7–10 days after number of moths in pheromone traps exceeds threshold; repeat after 3 weeks if necessary
	mildew	bupirimate	Add mancozeb or dithianon if risk of scab and weather wet, or use captan
	nutrition	calcium chloride	

Continue a 10-day programme of triadimefon until last round when replaced by bupirimate. Include dithianon or mancozeb or reduced rate of captan if scab control is required if weather wet. See product labels for dosage rates, but in many cases rates may be cut by 25% if crop is carefully monitored   Apply urea spray after harvesting to encourage leaves to rot and reduce risk of overwintering scab. Observe harvest interval following a spray application. NOTE: Do not treat apples between pink bud stage and the end of flowering. Choice of pesticide and use of mixtures will depend on severity of pest infestation.

(c) Cotton spray programme

Stage	Target	Treatment
Pre-sowing	grass weeds	Herbicide treatment. In some countries herbicide may be applied at sowing or later in the inter-row. Late applications may be needed, especially with mechanical harvesting.
At sowing	fungal disease	Fungicide seed treatment may be needed. In some countries an insecticide may also be applied to seed to protect against early season sucking pests (e.g. jassids).
First flower buds	non-Bt cotton	Start scouting for bollworms. Follow local recommendations (e.g. pyrethroid or alternative insecticide). Sprays may be needed at 7-day intervals until week 20 from germination, depending on pest infestation, rainfall and yield potential. Also scout for sucking pests and mites.
	Bt cotton	Scout, but sprays should only be required for sucking pests (e.g. aphids, whiteflies, and jassids).

Crop matures from about week 20 after germination.

Subtables (a) and (b) are from Matthews (1999).

In a crop, a spray will leave a pattern of droplets on the foliage and the ground under the plants, which will dry to form a surface deposit of the pesticide. If too high a volume is applied, the surplus liquid will drip from leaves and eventually increase the deposit on the soil. Although many have considered that high-volume spraying to be more effective as it is perceived to wet all surfaces, it can be very inefficient.

The deposit of pesticide active ingredient is then exposed to the effects of sunlight, rain and abrasion due to the movement of foliage. Some active ingredients are readily absorbed into the plants and may move systemically up through the plants and accumulate on the upper leaves. Some may move only across a leaf – translaminar – while some, like glyphosate, can be translocated downwards; thus, in the case of grasses the chemical reaches the rhizome. Deposits that remain on the leaf surface are effective by contact action or may be ingested by an insect, but remain the most exposed to degradation. Rain within 2 hours of a spray application could wash off a spray deposit, although the formulation is usually designed to stick the deposit on the foliage. Ultra-low volume oil-based sprays had the advantage of being more rain-fast. Very fine particles can adhere extremely well to surfaces. If the pesticide is too volatile, then loss of deposits by vapour lifting from the crop can occur. In some cases limited vapour action is useful as pests not in direct contact with a spray deposit may be killed, but downwind movement of pesticide vapour will cause environmental damage.

The development of some pesticides has aimed at increasing persistence; thus, the synthetic pyrethroids are more stable in sunlight than the natural pyrethrins. Nevertheless, the effectiveness of a deposit will decrease over time. One factor is the growth of the plants, which will increase the surface area of the foliage and thus dilute the impact of a deposit. Rapid plant growth in a crop such as cotton in the tropics required a weekly spray treatment during a sustained bollworm infestation. A low dose applied more frequently was more effective than attempting to apply a higher dose less often.

One of the factors on the label is the pre-harvest interval (PHI). This takes into account the persistence of the pesticide, the recommended dose, and environmental/climatic conditions to indicate the period over which a deposit will have decayed and no longer leave a residue above the MRL in the harvested produce. Thus, if a pest infestation is considered serious close to harvest, great care is needed to observe the PHI and to use a chemical that is considered suitable for applying close to harvest. This is a particular problem with crops such as lettuce which are eaten raw, and where a fungicide may be needed to prevent the fungal disease botrytis developing on the lettuce head between harvesting and being displayed in the marketplace.

Concentrations of pesticide solutions may also have upper limits imposed for safety. As volume rates decrease, the typical spray concentration used has increased, though regulators may specify an upper limit for some actives that are not to be exceeded. Fears of operator exposure and inhalation may increase with these changes and may need to be controlled.

This chapter has shown the wide range of equipment available for applying pesticides and the problems associated with determining when a pesticide should be applied.

References

Bache, D.H. and Johnstone, D.R. (1992) *Microclimate and Spray Dispersion*. Ellis Horwood, Chichester.

Butler Ellis, M.C., Swan, T. Miller, P.C.H., Waddelow, S., Bradley, A. and Tuck, C.R. (2002) Design factors affecting spray characteristics and drift performance of air induction nozzles. *Biosystems Engineering* **82**, 289–296.

Combellack, J.H. and Miller, P.C.H. (1999) A new twin fluid nozzle which shows promise for precision agriculture. *Proceedings, Brighton Crop Protection Conference – Weeds* 473–478.

De Snoo, G.R. and Luttik, R. (2004) Availability of pesticide-treated seed in arable fields. *Pest Management Science* **60**, 501–506.

Doble, S.J., Matthews, G.A., Rutherford, I. and Southcombe, E.S.E. (1985) A system for classifying hydraulic nozzles and other atomisers into categories of spray quality. *Proceedings, Brighton Crop Protection Conference – Weeds* II25-II33.

Holterman, H.J., van de Zande, J.C., Porskamp, H.A.J. and Huijsmans, J.F.M. (1997) Modelling spray drift from boom sprayers. *Computers and Electronics in Agriculture* **19**, 1–22.

Lodeman, E.G. (1896) *The Spraying of Plants*. Macmillan, London.

Matthews, G.A. (1999) *Application of Pesticides to Crops*. IC Press.

Matthews, G.A. (2000) *Pesticide Application Methods*. Third edition. Blackwell Scientific, Oxford.

Matthews, G.A. and Bateman, R.P. (2004) Classification criteria for fog and mist application of pesticides. *Aspects of Applied Biology* **71**, 55–60.

Matthews, G.A. and Thomas, N. (2000a) Working towards more efficient application of pesticides. *Pest Management Science* **56**, 974–976.

Matthews, G.A. and Thomas, N. (2000b) Effective use of air for low drift of fine sprays. *BCPC Symposium* **74**, 221–224.

Miller, P.C.H. (2003) The current and future role of application in improving pesticide use. *The BCPC International Congress* 247–254.

Murphy, S.D., Miller, P.C.H. and Parkin, C.S. (2000) The effect of boom section and nozzle configuration on the risk of spray drift. *Journal of Agricultural and Engineering Research* **75**, 127–137.

Phillips, J.C. and Miller, P.C.H. (1999) Field and wind tunnel measurements of the airborne spray volume downwind of single flat-fan nozzles. *Journal of Agricultural and Engineering Research* **72**, 161–170.

Piggott, S. and Matthews, G.A. (1999) Air induction nozzles: a solution to spray drift? *International Pest Control* **41**, 24–28.

Powell, E.S., Orson, J.H., Miller, P.C.H., Kudsk, P. and Mathiassen, S. (2003) Defining the size of target for air induction nozzles. *The BCPC International Congress* 267–272.

Robinson, T.H., Butler Ellis, C.M.C. and Power, J.D. (2003) Evaluation of nozzles for the application of a late fungicide spray. *The BCPC International Congress* 273–278.

Southcombe, E.S.E., Miller, P.C.H., Ganzelmeier, H., Van de Zande, J.C., Miralles, A. and Hewitt, A.J. (1997) The international (BCPC) spray classification system, including a drift potential factor. *Proceedings, Brighton Crop Protection Conference – Weeds* 371–380.

4 Operator exposure

Exposure to pesticides tends to be greatest for those who mix and apply the sprays in the field, especially those employed by contractors or who work on large estates and plantations where a pesticide may be applied on consecutive days and sometimes for a prolonged period during the year. Those preparing the spray are potentially at greatest risk of exposure to the concentrated pesticide product, whereas the applicator may be exposed only to the dilute spray. Worker exposure is therefore an important issue in occupational health, and is an essential part of the risk assessments in pesticide registration (van Hemmen and Brouwer, 1997). Operators can be exposed to pesticide that reaches the skin (dermal), by inhalation and by accidental ingestion (oral), for example by eating while working. The most important of these routes is dermal for commonly used pesticide application techniques.

Decisions on operator exposure are based on a comparison of the No Observed Adverse Effect Level (NOAEL) and an estimate of human exposure. The Acceptable Operator Exposure Level (AOEL) is derived from the NOAEL by dividing it by an assessment factor (usually by a factor of 100, which is essentially made up of two ×10 uncertainty factors (Anon, 1999a; Renwick, 1991) to allow for inter- and intra-species variation, as discussed in Chapter 2. In some countries, such as the USA, the margin of exposure (MOE) or margin of safety are derived in a similar manner. As it would be impossible to measure the exposure in all situations, there is considerable reliance on experimental data obtained from particular usage situations that have been incorporated into generic models such as the European Predictive Operator Exposure Model (EUROPOEM; Gilbert, 1995), which is still being developed.

Under the European approach to pesticide registration covered by Directive 91/414/EEC, this database can be used to estimate the amount of exposure for different situations (Glass *et al.*, 2000). Guidance on more general assessments of exposure to chemicals are given in the UK by the Interdepartmental Group on Health Risks from Chemicals (IGHRC) (Anon, 2004). Recognising the lack of accurate information from many countries, the World Health Organization (WHO) is collecting more information to improve knowledge of the extent and outcome of human exposure to pesticides, nationally, regionally and globally. WHO is also developing and providing tools for the collection of internationally harmonised data on human exposures to pesticides and more efficient collection, processing and analysis of information about pesticide products. The aim is to assist countries in capacity building for prevention and management of pesticide poisoning, and in decision-making for the safe management of pesticides. There is also a concern that studies on pesticide toxicology need to more relevant to occupational risk assessment (Ross *et al.*, 2001).

EUROPOEM will provide a tool for general exposure evaluation for use by member governments, but more data were required to test the validity of the predicted exposure level in different situations. Thus, field assessments have been carried out, especially in southern Europe (Machera *et al.*, 2001; Glass *et al.*, 2002b). The EUROPOEM database is available to be used in conjunction with existing models developed in the UK and Germany. In North America, a Pesticides Handlers Exposure Database (PHED) provides generic mixer/loader/applicator exposure data (Krieger, 1995). Work is being done to combine PHED and EUROPOEM datasets in a new North American model, the Agricultural Handlers Exposure Database (AHED) (van Hemmen and van der Jagt, 2005). Actual exposure will vary at different stages of the treatment process, depending on the type of pesticide product being applied (e.g. low concentration granule or a high concentrated liquid formulation), and on the handling and application procedures adopted. Thus, exposure data are usually independent of the active ingredient, but are affected by the formulation, packaging used and application equipment.

The impact of exposure will also be affected by the frequency of exposure. In Holland, the use of insecticides and fungicides was more frequent than the use of herbicides as they were used ten to twenty times a year on the most intensively treated crops, but single pesticide products were not used more than seven times a year (van Drooge *et al.*, 2001). In that study, ornamental crops such as chrysanthemums were treated more than arable crops. Some spray operators, such as those employed by contractors will be exposed for more days per year than individuals on small farms.

Potential *dermal exposure* is the total amount of pesticide landing on the body, including clothing, but the actual exposure of the skin will depend on the amount deposited directly on the skin plus any that penetrates clothing and is therefore available on the skin for absorption into the body. Operator exposure is significantly reduced by wearing protective clothing (Figs. 4.1 and 4.2). The basic requirement is good overalls of closely woven fabric. In temperate climates, impermeable materials are suitable and in many cases operators use disposable overalls made from a polypropylene material. Although this eliminates the need for laundering, such overalls are generally considered to be too hot to wear in tropical climates, and do not always provide as much protection as those made from cotton (Moreira *et al.*, 1999). Various special finishes to cotton fabrics have also been tried for use in tropical countries. Gilbert and Bell (1990) have described tests for the suitability of coveralls, but laboratory tests do not always provide an accurate indication of field performance (Glass *et al.*, 1998). Simulated wear studies have been conducted to assess the impact of treating garments with a fluoroalkyl

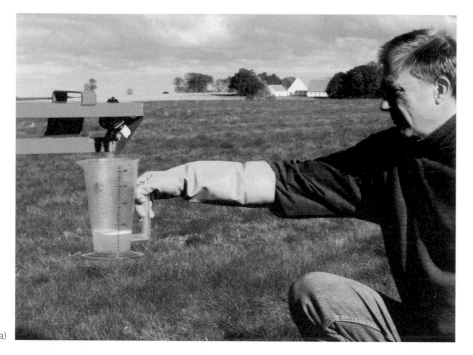

(a)

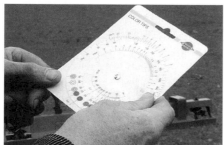

(b)

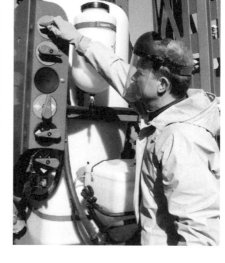

(c)

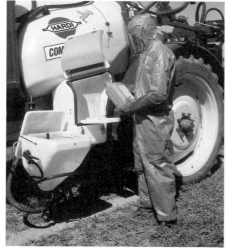

(d)

Fig. 4.1 Operating a sprayer. (a) Checking nozzle output with water; (b) examining nozzle calibration chart; (c) adjusting sprayer; (d) measuring pesticide. (*Continued.*)

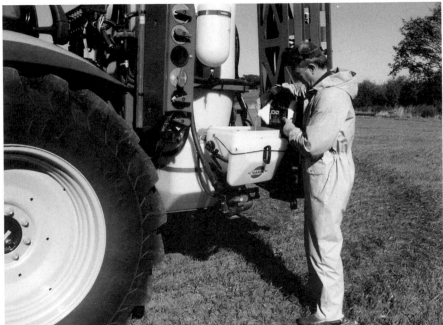

(e)

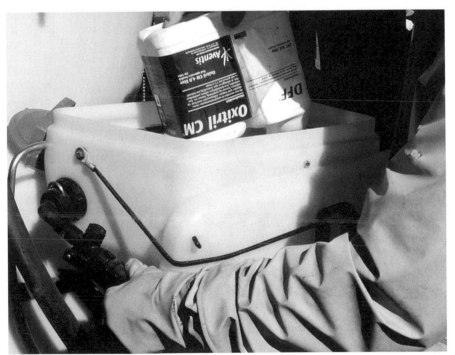

(f)

Fig. 4.1 (*Continued.*) (e) pouring pesticide into a low-level hopper; (f) rinsing containers (photographs from Hardi International). (*Continued.*)

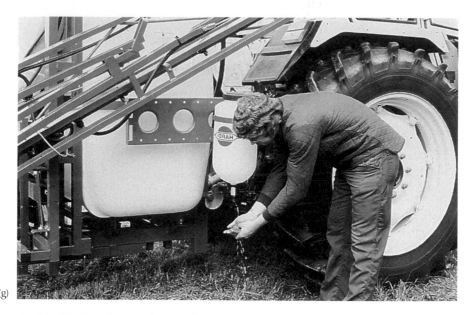

(g)

Fig. 4.1   (*Continued.*) (g) Washing hands.

methacrylate polymer in reducing sorption and penetration of a pesticide
(Shaw *et al.*, 1996). In further field studies, Shaw *et al.* (2000) reported that
cotton twill fabrics with and without a fluorochemical finish provide barrier
protection, as the amount of diluted spray which can penetrate the garment
is reduced. However, without the finish, the fabric absorbs the liquid and
will fail to provide protection once the fabric is saturated. These difficulties
with protective clothing emphasise the role of engineering control designs
to minimise – at source – the likelihood of any pesticide being on the sprayer
or leaking from it to – to subsequently contact the operator.

Laundering of garments does not always remove the entire pesticide
residue in a garment. Nelson *et al.* (1992) reported that the percentage not
removed can vary from 1% to over 40%. However, in the tropics some degradation will occur when the garments are exposed to sunlight (Shaw *et al.*,
1997). The washing of used protective clothing may also cross-contaminate
other garments.

Wearing an apron of impermeable plastic, especially when opening pesticide containers, will protect the overalls from splashing during preparation
of sprays and can be readily removed while spraying. Similarly, a face shield
is also recommended during mixing to protect the face, and especially the
eyes. Some countries prefer to recommend goggles but these do not protect
the face. When suitable overalls are not available or are too expensive for
small-scale farmers, the area of exposed skin should be minimised by wearing long trousers and a long-sleeved shirt. These need to be removed and
washed separately from domestic laundry as soon as possible after a spray
application has been completed. In Zimbabwe, many farmers fail to recognise

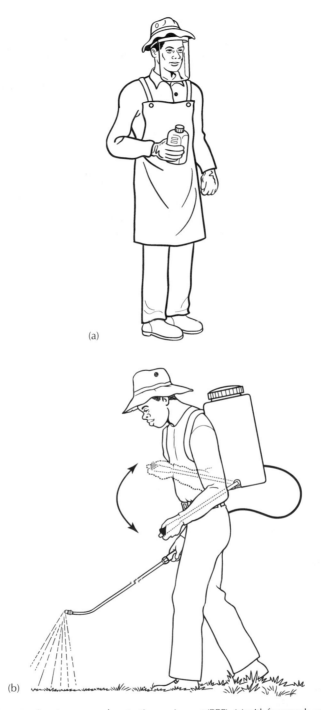

(a)

(b)

Fig. 4.2   Operator showing personal protective equipment (PPE): (a) with face mask, apron and gloves when preparing a spray; and (b) long-sleeved shirt, long trousers, hat and boots when operating a sprayer.

the colour coding on containers due to lack of training, and in consequence do not protect themselves (Maumbe *et al.*, 2003).

Inevitably, the *hands* are most likely to be exposed to sprays at all stages of application. Impermeable gloves are recommended, but generally these are uncomfortable to wear for prolonged periods. Their use is essential with the most hazardous pesticides, at least during the preparation of sprays and loading the sprayer, unless engineering controls (discussed later) provide sufficient protection. Poor glove hygiene and transfer to the skin or even the inside of the glove when removing and replacing gloves is a big problem. Once material is inside the glove the hydrated skin conditions may lead to increased absorption and higher amounts absorbed than if gloves had not been worn. Care is needed to avoid using contaminated gloves, so used gloves need to be washed. Where gloves are not used, there should always be a supply of water for washing any splashes off immediately. Even with gloves, the outer surface should be washed, to facilitate their removal without exposing a bare hand to pesticide. Larger sprayers are now fitted with a small extra water tank especially to allow the operator to wash gloves before removal, and to wash the hands.

Inhalation exposure is generally considered to be quite low compared with dermal exposure. This is because the amount of spray in the vicinity of the nose is generally low and the nose acts as an efficient filter such that only particles in the sub-10 µm range are likely to reach the lungs (respirable fraction). Studies on devices which aid in the passage of pharmaceuticals into the lungs for asthma control have shown that larger particles are trapped in the nose (Clay and Clarke, 1987), although some of these particles in the nasal cavity are often swallowed. The use of high-concentrate wettable or dispersible powders, which could puff into the operator's face, is less common, as they have largely been replaced by wettable granules, or the dry formulation has been packaged into plastic sachets that break up and expose the contents to water. The main concern with inhalation exposure is when pesticides are applied as fogs, where a high proportion of the droplets are below 25 µm. It is essential to wear the correct respiratory protection equipment (RPE) when fogging, especially inside buildings. The main item is a respirator, which has a filter to remove the very small particles of pesticide in a fog. The correct filter, depending on the chemical being applied, must be fitted and replaced according to instructions. Inexpensive disposable masks are not respirators and often merely reduce the impaction of spray droplets directly on the skin around the nose and mouth. Some more expensive protectors which cover the operator's head may not be true respirators but have a pump to draw air through the filter and blow the filtered air over the face.

The *feet* should always be well protected by wearing 'rubber' boots or equivalent, with the bottom of the trouser legs placed over the boot so that liquid or granules do not fall into the boot. In some areas spray operators fail to wear shoes, but if they do so the shoes are often of very poor quality and made from absorbent materials.

The *ears* should always be protected when the noise of the operating spraying equipment exceeds 85 decibels. This applies especially to manually carried motorised equipment fitted with a two-stroke engine, and when pulsejet fogging equipment is used.

Methodology of measuring exposure

One of the earliest methods of assessing potential dermal exposure was to attach absorbent cotton pads to different parts of the body (Durham and Wolfe, 1962). The amount of pesticide collected on seven to sixteen pads was determined and related to the area of relevant part of the body (Table 4.1). The hands are more frequently covered with cotton gloves. Exposure was usually reported as mg of pesticide per hour of application, although some studies report in mg per litre of spray applied. Absorbent pads and gloves will hold a greater volume of spray than the bare skin, but have the advantage of accumulating spray over a long period of a spray application. Placing the pads and cotton gloves under the overalls and impermeable gloves can assess the validity of protective clothing. Significant exposure can occur at the interface of a garment and skin, for example around the neck and cuffs (Anon, 2002).

Pads are typically only 26 cm^2, but some are 100 cm^2 (10 cm × 10 cm), and so represent a small fraction of the surface to which they are attached. Another early method was to use a strip of film placed at different parts of the body (Fig. 4.3a) (Tunstall and Matthews, 1965). Colour dyes have been used (Fig. 4.3b) to show where the spray was collected on the body. The main alternative to the pads is for the spray operator to wear a disposable overall (Chester and Ward, 1983; Sutherland *et al.*, 1990; Chester, 1995; Machera *et al.*, 2002). This can subsequently be cut into small sections, each of which is analysed separately. These studies can be performed using a tracer dye (often

Table 4.1   Areas of different parts of an adult body

Body part	Area (cm^2)	% of total body area
Hands	900	4.5
Arms	2,700	13.5
Head and neck	1,200	6
Front of body	3,800	19
Back of body	3,800	19
Thighs	3,800	19
Legs and feet	3,800	19
Total	20,000	100

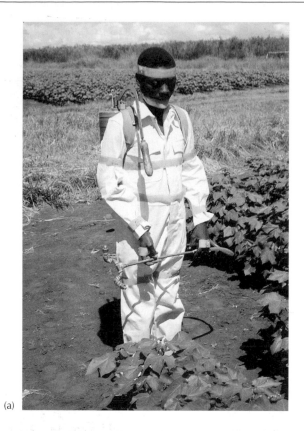

(a)

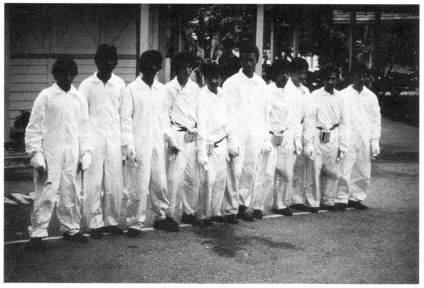

(b)

Fig. 4.3 Measuring operator exposure. (a) Early experiment with 35 mm film used as a collecting surface attached to different parts of the body to collect coloured dye. (b) A team of operators at a plantation, showing dye mostly on lower legs after applying a coloured dye in a herbicide. (*Continued.*)

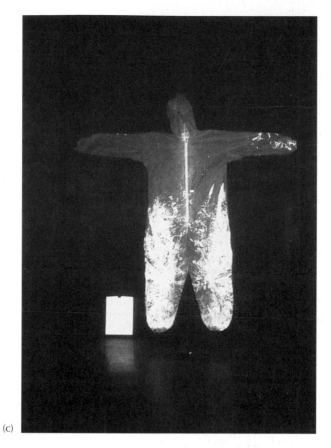

(c)

Fig. 4.3   (*Continued.*) (c) Fluorescent dye on overalls (photographs GAM, ICI and NRI).

a fluorescent dye) so that the distribution of chemical in different areas can be assessed visually before quantitative analysis (Fig. 4.3c). Special apparatus using a dodecahedron of ultra-violet lights to visualise fluorescent deposits on clothing (Roff, 1994) has been developed. Using fluorescent tracers, video imaging and pads, Fenske (1990) reported a non-uniform distribution of spray deposits, which were dependent upon work activity and the method of application. The highest deposits were recorded on the lower part of the forearms of those preparing sprays.

In assessing the surface area of a person, the 'rule of nines' is also used (Fig. 4.4). This assumes that the head, front and rear upper and lower torso, each arm and each leg are all approximately 9% of the total body area. With smaller children (aged 5+ years) the head is about 15%, each arm 9.5%, each leg 17%, and the front and back torso each 16%, while for a one-year-old toddler the head is again proportionally larger.

Regulatory authorities use data obtained from EUROPOEM and similar sources to estimate the exposure of operators when using particular products

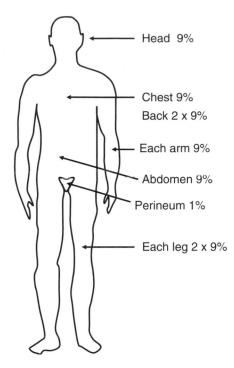

Head 9%

Chest 9%
Back 2 x 9%

Each arm 9%

Abdomen 9%

Perineum 1%

Each leg 2 x 9%

Fig. 4.4   The 'rule of nines'. This is used primarily for a quick assessment of the area of the body affected by burns; it is also useful in assessing coverage of the body by spray.

and equipment. Examples of the types of analysis for a tractor and knap-sack sprayer are shown in Table 4.2. Refinement of the extent of exposure is dependent on more information on how the pesticide is actually used (Hamey, 2001).

In vineyard spraying, the use of a hooded or 'tunnel' sprayer reduced operator exposure compared to use of an air-assisted with a centrifugal fan (Coffman *et al.*, 1999).

Exposure of hands

The hands, inevitably, are the part of the body most exposed to pesticides, due to handling of containers and when operating equipment. Data from PHED indicates that a person mixing and loading pesticide in the USA can be exposed to 6300 µg/kg ai when not wearing gloves compared to only 51.1 µg/kg ai when wearing gloves (Fenske and Day, 2005). The type of exposure will depend on many factors, but in the worst case the whole hand could be coated with liquid. Substances can be removed from the surface of the skin (especially the hands) by using swabs or towels, moistened with a solvent, such as 95% ethanol. The technique does not indicate what could

Table 4.2 Example of an estimate of operator exposure. (This example is to show the procedure in principle. The extent of operator exposure will vary with different equipment and the extent of operator training and care taken in practice.)

	Tractor sprayer with hydraulic nozzles	Knapsack sprayer
Product concentration	250 mg/ml	250 mg/ml
Concentration in use	0.5 mg/ml	0.5 mg/ml
Spray volume	200 l/ha	225 l/ha#
Work rate	50 ha/day	1 ha/day
Number of tank loads	20/day	15/day
Contamination of hand	0.01 ml	3.3 ml*
Per mixing operation, so with gloves	0.2 ml/day	49.5 ml/day
5% reaches the skin	0.01 ml/day	2.475 ml/day
During spraying over	5 h	8 h
Contamination of body	10 ml/h [6.5 ml on hands, 1.0 ml on body, 2.5 ml on legs]	50 ml/h [10 ml on hands, 15 ml on body, 25 ml on legs##]
With overalls, no gloves	34.6 ml/day	116 ml/day [assumes 100% reaches the skin on unprotected hands, but 5% on body and 15% on legs##]
Absorbed dose during mixing with gloves	0.25 mg/day [0.01 × 250 × 0.1**]	61.88 mg/day [2.475 × 250 ×0.1**]
Without gloves	5 mg/day [0.2 × 250 ×0.1**]	1237.5 mg/day [49.5 × 250 × 0.1**]
During application	1.73 mg/day [34.6 × 0.5 ×0.1**]	5.8 mg/day [116 × 0.5 × 0.1**]
Inhalation exposure	0.01 ml/h	0.01 ml/h
Inhalation absorbed dose	0.025 mg/day [0.01 ×5 × 0.5]	0.04 mg/day 100% absorption
Thus, total predicted exposure	2.01 mg/day [0.25 + 1.73 + 0.025] with PPE	67.72 mg/day
(which is for a person weighing 60 kg	0.033 mg/kg bw/day	1.128 mg/kg bw/day) [This last value is compared with the AOEL of the pesticide being applied]

If NOAEL is 800 mg/kg bw/day, then a systemic AOEL would be set at 0.8 mg/kg bw/day. If total systemic exposure (i.e. the absorbed dose) was estimated at 0.03 mg/kg bw/day, this is 4% of the AOEL, whereas 1.128 is 141%, and not acceptable. If with the knapsack, through improved glove performance/hygiene the amount reaching the skin is lowered to 1%, this reduces the exposure to 0.31 mg/kg bw/day (i.e. 39% of AOEL).

*This value is based on a trial with small-scale farmers asked to measure out a dye solution with a small 50-ml plastic cup (Craig and Mbevi, 1993). Different techniques of dispensing small quantities can significantly reduce operator exposure; for example use of tablet formulation, water-soluble sachets and containers with built-in measures.

**This assumes 10% absorption through the skin.

This is 15 knapsack loads.

These values are used for illustration and may differ according to circumstances.

have been absorbed before the skin was washed. Some laboratory tests to assess exposure of hands were conducted by Cinalli *et al.* (1992) with different liquids. Using three non-aqueous liquids, subjects were asked to wipe their hands with a cloth saturated in liquid. They then used a weighed dry cloth to wipe their hands and the amount removed was determined by the weight gained on the dry cloth. Unfortunately, the dry cloth may not remove all that was on the surface of the hands, especially from between the fingers or under the nails. These authors also determined how much was retained on hands by immersion in a container of the liquid and weighing the container before and after immersion. Using a similar immersion technique with water containing a surfactant, Matthews (2001) reported that a bare dry hand retained on average 0.0045 ml/cm^2, whereas there was no significant increase if the hand was already wet. Excess liquid dripped off, depending on the position of the hand and movement. Less water was retained on the surface of a vinyl glove. The EPA generally estimates that a man would have 6 ml retained on a hand.

To protect hands, the wearing of impermeable gloves is recommended, but these vary in their thickness and suitability, especially when adjusting small parts such as nozzles. Gloves with a cuff long enough to be covered by the end of the coverall sleeve are advised so that any liquid, or granule, that is on the arm does not pass down inside the glove. Neoprene and nitrile gloves provide protection to a range of solvents and oils, and are suitable when using emulsifiable concentrate and similar liquid formulations. Nevertheless, users should wash off any pesticide as soon as possible as some chemicals can penetrate a glove. Care is needed when washing gloves, as the rinsate subsequently acts as a source of exposure for other workers or family members, water courses, etc. Often, contamination of the gloves occurs when the operator removes the gloves using a clean hand to remove a dirty glove. Washing the gloves before removal is advised, but care is still needed when removing the glove. In some situations, especially in the tropics, an impermeable glove causes the hand to sweat and this may increase the risk of absorption. Spray operators not using gloves should only apply the less hazardous pesticides and have a bucket of water readily available so that a bare hand that has been exposed to spray can be washed immediately. Access to water for washing was shown to be beneficial among workers in Kenya (Ohayo-Mitoko *et al.*, 1999).

One major cause of exposure to hands was due to the old style of metal container, which had a lip around the edge. Concentrate often collected on the top of a drum after it had been tilted to pour out liquid into a measure or directly into a spray tank. This type of drum was considered to be a major factor among farmers who suffered pesticide poisoning when dipping sheep. Farmers may have used the drum as many as eight times a day to top-up the dip tank. This problem has been overcome in the new design of containers. On small farms in the tropics and for amateur gardeners, pesticides have often been measured using the container cap (Craig and Mbevi, 1993; Harrington *et al.*, 2005). In one series of tests, the spray concentration varied from 55 to 177% of the intended concentration, a fault that can be reduced when sachets with the correct dose for one sprayer load are used. Another factor is the amount of residue, with up to 31 mg of the active substance being left in the container cap. This method of measuring inevitably results in the operator being exposed to the concentrate, as few wear gloves. In the home garden situation, exposure of the operator to diluted spray was typically 20 ml/h, with up to 10 mg/h of the active substance, while a single spraying operation lasted from 5 to 15 minutes (Harrington *et al.*, 2005).

In order to reduce the need for personal protective clothing, emphasis has been placed on engineering controls to minimise exposure.

Inhalation exposure

In the open air, the risk of inhaling spray droplets is extremely low. Most sprays contain only a small fraction of the volume in droplets smaller than 100 µm. While these small droplets can shrink, especially on hot days and with low humidity, the smallest droplets in the range of 1–10 µm that could be inhaled are readily carried downwind and away from the spray operator. Any larger droplets close to the nose may be deposited on the face or filtered within the nose, and would not reach the lungs. The situation is different when applying pesticides inside buildings, stores and glasshouses where small droplets can remain airborne close to the operator.

Protection from small airborne droplets (<25 µm diameter) is necessary when fogging. A respirator is then essential, with suitable filters to remove the small droplets. Care is needed that the filters are still effective and, if there is any doubt, new filters suitable for the pesticide being used should be fitted. Disposable face-masks are not respirators and are only useful if dusts are applied with larger particles or the operator wishes to reduce dermal exposure in the vicinity of the mouth and nose.

Inhalation exposure studies

Exposure to airborne spray is ideally checked out using personal monitors, which have a pump system to draw air through a filter (Wolfe, 1976). The filter may be a simple cotton gauze or adsorbent resin. In both cases it is important to know the breathing rate of the person and the volume of air sampled in order to interpret the potential inhalation of a pesticide. Personal monitors mounted in the breathing zone of an operator are calibrated to have a flow of 1–2 litres of air per minute. Bjugstad and Torgrimsen (1996), using a respiration rate of 1.75 m³/h, calculated exposure when using several types of application equipment in a greenhouse. The highest respiratory exposure was, as expected, when using a thermal fogger, hence the need for using RPE. In pest control operations by professionals, airborne concentrations of permethrin were highest when dusts were applied, especially when treatment was above the operators, and when several worked together in a confined area (Llewellyn *et al.*, 1996).

Biomonitoring

Assessments of exposure determine how much reaches a person and, depending upon the extent to which the body is covered by clothing, how much is actually on the skin. Human skin protects the body very effectively from chemicals, especially in relation to the skin of other animals such as rats, but inevitably a proportion will be absorbed through the skin and reach the bloodstream. The pesticide, like other chemicals in the body, will reach the liver and be subject to breakdown, with metabolites being excreted via the kidney. To determine how much has entered the body, the normal practice is to analyse urine samples. Some biomonitoring studies have been carried out with a low-toxicity pesticide and its metabolites measured in urine samples (e.g. Krieger and Dinoff, 2000). Skin moisture will affect absorption, as indicated by increased dermal absorption of propoxur under conditions of high humidity and 30°C temperature (Meuling *et al.*, 1997).

When studying the impact of dipping sheep in an organophosphate (OP) pesticide, urine samples from sheep dippers pre- and post-dipping were compared with those of office workers and others (Table 4.3). The low level of urinary metabolites in those with no known occupational exposure may be due to domestic use or from dietary sources (Nutley *et al.*, 1995). Total pesticide OP metabolites in samples from a person who made an unsuccessful suicide attempt were 1000-fold higher than those from sheep dippers. Most exposure was due to the concentrate; thus, 100 µl of concen-

Table 4.3 Urinary dialkyl phosphate data from various occupational groups and workers (adapted from Nutley *et al.*, 1995)

Occupation	Mean (range) total urinary 'ethyl' phosphate metabolites (nmol/mmol creatine)	90% results less than	No. of samples/ individuals
Office workers	1.6 (0–32)	6	106/106
Sheep dippers			
Pre-dipping	5.6 (9–162)	14	159/159
Post-dipping	15 (0–189)	40	337/167
Agricultural workers			
Pre-exposure	1.3 (0–17)	5	35/35
Post-exposure	10.3 (0–159)	27	59/35
Formulators	42.8 (0–479)	72	88/10

trate would be equivalent to exposure to 150 ml of the diluted pesticide in the dip. Unfortunately, very few of those workers dipping sheep wore the recommended protective clothing (Buchanan *et al.*, 2001), with many considering that it was not possible to wear the clothing while handling the sheep. Inhalation was only a minor route of exposure.

Studies with diazinon showed that 40% of the OP was excreted during the first 24 hours, after which the rate slowed to about 5% per day between days 3 and 7 (Wester *et al.*, 1993; Anon, 1999b). In Spain, urine samples from operators exposed to the insecticide acetamiprid applied with a spray gun in greenhouses also showed that excretion was primarily within 24 hours (Marin Juan *et al.*, 2004) (Fig. 4.5). Similarly, in tests with the OP propetamphos, a urinary metabolite was shown to be a suitable biomarker, with excretion over a longer period following dermal compared to oral exposure (Garfitt *et al.*, 2002).

Paraquat is very suitable for bio-monitoring as it is not metabolised, and it is rapidly and completely excreted via the kidneys, remaining comparatively stable in urine samples. Overall, where assessments have been made, the paraquat concentration in urine was low, with the majority of samples being below the limit of detection. According to Wester and Maibach (1985), paraquat is only minimally absorbed, especially in comparison with other commonly available pesticides. None of the samples contained paraquat at levels which would be indicative of a risk of poisoning (Table 4.4). Nevertheless, the importance of good quality equipment that does not leak cannot be overemphasised to reduce operator exposure to dilute pesticide over a prolonged period. Similarly, no adverse health effects were to be expected following biomonitoring of acetochlor, although tractor drivers using open cabs were more exposed than those who had a closed cab (Gustin *et al.*, 2005).

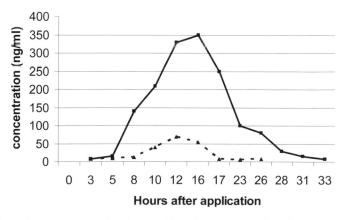

Fig. 4.5 Biomonitoring urine samples, showing effect of wearing PPE (adapted from Marin Juan, A. *et al.* (2004), *Aspects of Applied Biology* **71**, 405–408). Solid line without PPE; dotted line with PPE.

Table 4.4   Worker exposure and absorption of paraquat (adapted from Lock and Wilks, 2001)

Country	Application method	Spray dilution (%w/v)	Dermal exposure (mg/h)	Inhalation exposure (mg/h)	Urine level (mg/l)
Malaysia	Hand-held	0.1–0.2	<0.01–12[a]	0–0.005	<0.05–0.76
Sri Lanka	Hand-held	0.03–0.04	0.94–2.7[b$]	<0.03	
Costa Rica	Hand-held	0.1–0.2	0.2–5.7	0–0.043	<0.03–0.24
USA	Hand-held	0.2	0.01–0.57[a]	<0.001	<0.02
	Vehicle-mounted	0.1	0.01–3.4[a] 12–170[b]	0–0.002	<0.02
	Vehicle-mounted	0.05–0.1	7.0–42[a] 12–169[b]	0–0.07	<0.02–0.03
	Aerial	0.3	0.1–2.4[b+] 0.05–0.26[b#]	0–0.047[+] 0–0.06	

[a], Exposure to uncovered skin; [b], total dermal exposure; [+], aerial – flagger; [#], aerial – pilot; [$], mg/g paraquat sprayed.

Biomonitoring has been used to assess the exposure of persons using small application devices inside residences, where exposures are considerably less and occur over a longer period than in open-field agricultural use (Kreiger *et al.*, 2001). Generally, measurements indicate exposure more accurately as they reflect the extent of dermal absorption through the skin over the whole body and the effect of excretion of the pesticide. In addition to urinary monitoring, the possibility of using saliva samples to monitor exposure to some pesticides has been considered (Denovan *et al.*, 2000; Fenske and Day, 2005).

Other sources of information on assessing pesticide exposure include the reviews by Chester (1993), Curry *et al.* (1995), and the International Centre for Pesticides and Health Risk Prevention, a Collaborating Centre on Occupational Health, specialising in pesticides, which is based in Milan, and publishes a newsletter, *Pesticide Safety News*, in English, Italian and Spanish.

First aid

If a spray operator becomes ill, while working, the doctor must be informed of the name of the active ingredient and given as much information as possible by being shown a leaflet or label about the chemical being used. Treatment by a doctor will depend very much on the type of poisoning. When using an OP or a carbamate (anticholinesterase), an injection of atropine is useful, but suitable antidotes for organochlorine poisoning are not available. A person who has ingested liquid that contained paraquat can be treated by their ingesting large quantities of Fuller's earth, which adsorbs the herbicide. Morphine should not be given to patients affected by pesticide poisoning.

A first-aid kit and a supply of clean water for drinking and washing any contaminated areas of the body should be readily available. On large-scale spraying programmes first-aid kits should be carried in vehicles and aircraft. People regularly involved in applying OP pesticides should undergo routine medical examinations in order to check cholinesterase levels in their blood plasma.

The Department of Labor and Industries in Washington State, USA, implemented a cholinesterase monitoring rule in 2004 and 2005. Thresholds for monitoring were written into the rule at 50 hours in a 30-day period during 2004, and this has been reduced to 30 hours in a 30-day period for 2005, when working with OP and *N*-methyl carbamate insecticides. The rule may be amended as more information is obtained. During 2004, baseline tests were carried out on 2630 employees, and 580 underwent further monitoring. Of these 580 employees 16.7% had a 20% or more depression of enzyme levels, necessitating the employer to evaluate pesticide handling practices. Twenty-two employees were removed from exposure because the red blood cell cholinesterase depression was equal to or exceeded 30%, or the plasma cholinesterase depression was ≥40%, but three of these workers had used the pesticides for 30–50 hours, while two reported less than 30 hours, use (Anon, 2005). The number of hours for which the remaining 2050 employees in the baseline survey were exposed to the insecticides was not indicated. This monitoring was not linked to any specific pesticide, application method or crop being treated, but some of the poisonings occurred following the use of tractor-mounted air-blast orchard sprayers. Irrespective of the cause of poisoning, these findings emphasise the importance of engineering controls to minimise exposure and the use of the correct protective clothing. Moreover, they also indicate the problems associated with using the most highly toxic insecticides.

In many countries there are dedicated poisons centres from which medical doctors can obtain advice on treatment. In contrast, some tropical countries lack the expertise (Ngowi *et al.*, 2001a), yet it is in these countries that some of the most toxic pesticides are used, often with poor-quality sprayers that leak, and by untrained operators. Thus, occupational poisoning has continued to be a serious problem among farm-workers, for example, those in the coffee-growing areas of Tanzania (Ngowi *et al.*, 2001b).

Periods of exposure

Spray preparation

Most pesticides are applied as sprays, so the main concern is when the concentrate is diluted to prepare a spray. In the past, many problems occurred when opening containers and pouring pesticide due to 'glugging' and splashing, but significant changes in container design have improved the ease of pouring pesticides. Containers larger than 1 litre usually have a standard thread opening of external 64 mm diameter.

Concern about operators climbing up on to a tractor or vehicle-mounted sprayer tank to pour concentrate from drums into the tank opening has led to the design and adoption of low-level induction bowls that must be no higher than 1 m above the ground. The induction bowl makes it easier for operators to add the spray concentrate, and as they are fitted with rinsing nozzles, the empty containers can be thoroughly washed (triple rinsed) before disposal. Studies have confirmed that spillages were reduced by using the induction bowl, which is now used on 82% of the arable area of the UK (Garthwaite, 2002).

Widespread adoption of low-level induction bowls has undoubtedly facilitated transfer of the formulation into a sprayer. Glass *et al.* (2002a) reported that usually less than 0.01 ml per fill of the sprayer was on the operator, when pouring pesticide from a container into an induction hopper. The use of an apron and face-shield at this stage can avoid splashes on the coveralls or face. There is little risk of creating small droplets which could be inhaled during mixing and loading, so inhalation exposure is minimal (Wolf *et al.*, 1999).

Many engineering control measures are now available on the modern sprayer. Drain plugs are remotely activated, while hydraulic lifting and folding of booms, freely draining tank surfaces, bayonet-fitted nozzles and remote controls are just some items that have contributed enormously to reducing exposure levels for operators.

Further reductions of operator exposure are possible with the adoption of closed-transfer systems (Glass *et al.*, 2002b), with initial tests with liquid formulations having shown significant decreases in the amount of liquid that is collected on the hands and overalls (Table 4.5) (Glass *et al.*, 2004).

Ideally, the pesticide is transferred to the sprayer by a closed-transfer system, incorporating a measure, that meets the BS 6356 Part 9. So far, these closed-transfer systems have been used for specialist or certain high-volume uses (Fig. 4.6). Many pesticides are not available in suitable containers, with

Table 4.5 Volume of liquid (ml) from field studies when using induction bowl or a closed-transfer system

	Mean value*	Maximum value
Induction bowl		
Body	0.07	0.65
Hands	0.25	1.05
Closed-transfer system		
Body	0.01	0.03
Hands	0.03	0.06

*Minimum values were below the level of detection.

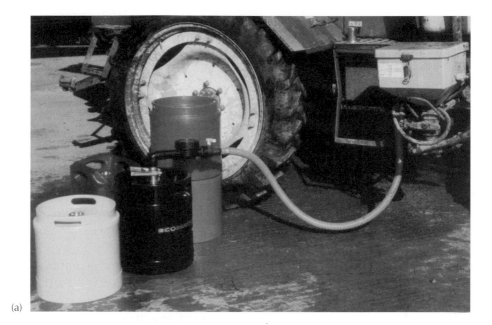

(a)

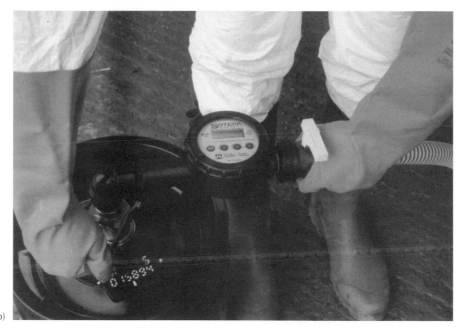

(b)

Fig. 4.6 Closed-transfer system. (a) Showing drum connected to sprayer. (b) Close up of drum with operator attaching it to sprayer.

the chemical industry appearing reluctant to support multi-trip containers in many countries due to cost implications. The provision of different formulations, including wettable granules as well as liquids, makes it difficult for a standard system to be developed. However, some closed-transfer systems do fit standard containers, and allow the empty container to be washed out.

During spraying

In large-scale agriculture, the operator is well protected inside the tractor cab, but must be careful not to take contaminated clothing into the cab, which is supplied with filtered air. In a well-designed cab, filters remove at least 99% of the aerosol particles larger than 3 μm (Hall *et al.*, 2002). Care is needed if nozzles, the spray boom or other components need attention, when the hands in particular could be exposed to concentrated spray deposits. Touching surfaces in the cab then transfers pesticide to the steering wheel and seats (Landers, 2004). Most sprayers now have a separate water tank for washing any spray off the gloves, and separate lockers for clean and used PPE. Actual exposure during this period should therefore be minimal, although the period during which the operator may be exposed can be several hours. Even when approved coveralls are used, the correct wearing of the protective clothing is an important factor determining its protective value to the wearer, as demonstrated by research sponsored by the Health and Safety Executive in the UK (HSE, 2002).

In many parts of southern Europe and elsewhere and in glasshouses, the traditional method of high-volume spraying has continued. In Holland, typically a motorised pump was used to feed spray along a flexible hose at high pressure (often 20–30 bar) to a manually directed 'pistol'. Spray volumes usually exceed 1000 litres per hectare. A second person may assist with moving the long hose. The operator may walk into the area treated and can be covered with spray. Data (Table 4.6) from de Vreede *et al.* (1998), with a period of about 9 minutes for mixing and loading followed by an average of 81 minutes for application, confirmed that the hands were the most exposed part of the body, especially during mixing and loading of the sprayer. Of all their samples ($n = 190$), mean penetration through the overalls was on average less than 5%. Walking backwards away from the spray reduced exposure by a factor of 7. Operator exposure was also considerably reduced

Table 4.6 Mean amounts of active substance (mg/h) detected on spray operators using high volume application (geometric standard deviation)

Source of exposure	Mean	GSD
Inhalation	5.1	(5.0)
Gloves (mixing/loading)	13,110	(7.1)
Gloves (application)	760	(4.9)
Overalls	1,710	(3.1)
Underwear	40	(4.4)
Socks	7.5	(3.3)

when a small vehicle- or trolley-mounted sprayer was used instead of the long hose (Nuyttens *et al.*, 2004) (Fig. 4.7).

On small farms with manually carried equipment the situation is quite different. This is especially true in tropical countries, where relatively few farmers can afford to use PPE and find it uncomfortable in a hot climate, even when applying highly toxic pesticides. Many operators have had only primary education or are illiterate, and so have little knowledge about the pesticides they are applying (Mekonnen and Agonafir, 2002). Operators are not only exposed to the diluted spray for lengthy periods as they tend to walk through crops with the spray nozzle held in front of them, but poor quality equipment and lack of maintenance often also results in leaks of pesticide over the operator's hands and back. The FAO has issued minimum requirements for sprayers in an effort to develop better quality equipment (see http://www.fao.org/docrep/X2244E/X2244E00.htm). Even among professional pest control operators using small equipment, including compression sprayers, the highest contamination resulted from the use of leaking application equipment (Llewellyn *et al.*, 1996).

Early studies indicated that placing the nozzle behind the operator would significantly reduce exposure to pesticides (Fernando, 1956; Tunstall and Matthews, 1965), but few farmers have accepted this. The exposure of an

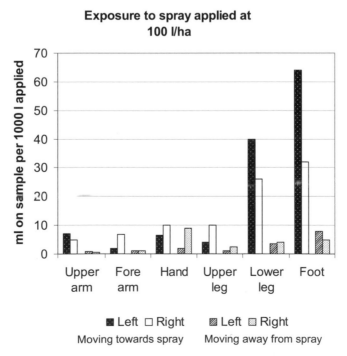

Fig. 4.7 Contrast when moving towards and away from the spray (adapted from Nuyttens, D. *et al.* (2004), *Aspects of Applied Biology* **71**, 349–356).

operator, walking through growing cotton with a knapsack and with the lance held in front of their body – as most operators do – is on the lower legs. This exposure could be reduced by holding the lance downwind of the operator as recommended with the spinning disc sprayer (Table 4.7) (Thornhill *et al.*, 1996). The spinning disc sprayer applies a higher concentration of spray, but the volume applied is far lower and the person holding the sprayer does not walk through treated foliage. Thus, the net exposure shown in Table 4.7 (c) is similar to that indicated in Table 4.7 (a) with the lance held downwind.

In Argentina, operators using a knapsack sprayer were exposed to 78 ml/h and 12 ml/h for treating Swiss chard and lettuce crops respectively, with most pesticide found on the lower legs and gloves (Hughes *et al.*, 2004).

Operators of manually carried equipment are often exposed to spillages and leaks from sprayer tanks and trigger valves, especially if the sprayers are poorly maintained. Farmers often complain that spare parts are difficult to obtain so they contrive to repair sprayers with inappropriate materials. There is a raised flange on the side of the tank closest to the straps on some sprayers to protect the operator from spillages from the sprayer. In some countries, a simple plastic tabard has been supplied to reduce direct exposure of the body yet provide adequate ventilation. Protection of the legs and feet was required for users of knapsack sprayers applying the herbicide paraquat, as most potential dermal exposure was on these areas of the body (Machado-Neto *et al.*, 1998).

Ohayo-Mitoko *et al.* (1999) reported in Kenya that acetylcholinesterase inhibition was greater in those workers spraying compared to mixers, presumably because they were exposed over longer periods. The study also

Table 4.7   Potential operator exposure with a lever-operated knapsack sprayer in cotton: (a) holding the lance downwind; (b) in front of the operator; and (c) a spinning disc VLV sprayer (ULVA+) holding lance downwind. Data are from Thornhill *et al.* (1996)

Part of body	Area of disposable overall (cm^2)	Deposit (a) (μl/l)	Deposit (b) (μl/l)	Deposit (c) (μl/l)
Hood (head)	1,200	1.8	45.6	9.3
Mask	172	0.7	3.2	0.05
Right arm	1,350	29.7	322.5	63.1
Left arm	1,350	76.3	191.0	133.0
Gloves (hand)	900	23.6	269.4	33.6
Right leg	1,250	62.7	444.3	11.9
Left leg	1,250	42.6	416.2	21.3
Right thigh	1,900	52.6	413.3	13.1
Left thigh	1,900	45.9	383.2	6.1
Front torso	2,750	60.9	209.3	33.9
Rear torso	2,750	26.2	45.7	30.4
Front abdomen	3,550	25.0	477.4	39.7
Rear abdomen	3,550	38.0	139.7	65.8
Total	23,872	486.0	3,360.8	461.25

confirmed that workers using WHO Class III pesticides were less affected than those spraying more toxic pesticides.

The exposure of those who wear only a long-sleeved shirt and long trousers, or the equivalent local clothing, can be minimised by controlling the spray pressure. Operator exposure was reduced by using a control flow valve that controlled the pressure to avoid either a too-fine or a too-coarse spray (Shaw *et al.*, 2000). Applying a more coarse spray from an air-induction nozzle can also reduce operator exposure (Wicke *et al.*, 1999).

In semi-arid areas, ULV spraying has been extensively adopted on cotton, although more recently to follow IPM, there has been a change to very low volume (VLV), generally about 10 l/ha using water-based formulations, as this allowed more choice of insecticide. With the application of highly toxic ULV formulations, a study by Kummer and van Sittert (1986), confirmed by biomonitoring, indicated an increased absorption of insecticides, though no clinical signs or symptoms of intoxication were observed. Most exposure occurred while the sprayer was being filled from the containers.

After spraying

Care is also needed after spraying. Any of the unused pesticide product must be returned to the store, and all equipment must be washed after use, otherwise residues will accumulate and quantities subsequently washed off may be harmful if they enter a watercourse (Ramwell *et al.*, 2004). By careful calibration, all of the dilute spray will have been used as the treatment of a field is being completed, so washing of the tank can be done within the treated field. By having extra water available in the field, the washings of the sprayer tank can be applied by spraying on the last swath. In some countries where diluted pesticide-contaminated water must be disposed of, special areas known as 'biobeds' are used (Fogg and Carter, 1998; Henriksen *et al.*, 2003; Basford *et al.*, 2004) (Fig. 4.8). One type of biobed consists of a lined pit filled with a mixture of 50% straw, 25% peat and 25% soil and covered with turf grass. Fogg *et al.* (2003a) reported that biobeds offered a viable means of degrading some mixtures of herbicides and insecticides, although it may be necessary to avoid releasing certain pesticides to a biobed. Water management is crucial with lined beds to ensure sufficient moisture for microbial degradation, yet avoid overflow from the bed. With unlined beds, the most mobile pesticides were liable to leaching, although >99% was removed by the system and degraded within 9 months (Fogg *et al.*, 2003b). Pesticide detected in drainage from a biobed was 0.1% of that caused by run-off from a concrete surface. Farm-scale effluent treatment plants can also used to remove small quantities of pesticides from water (Harris *et al.*, 1991).

Traditionally, farmers have disposed most of their waste in on-farm dumps and by burning packaging where possible, but the Agricultural Waste Regulations, which come into force in 2005, will affect the way that

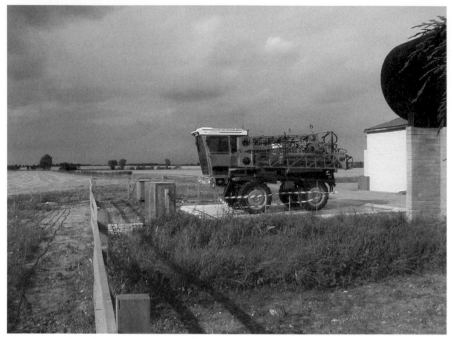

Fig. 4.8   Washing the sprayer on a bunded area draining into a biobed in the foreground (photograph W. Basford).

farmers can manage their waste, unless they can obtain the necessary permits or licences. In general, they will have to use licensed waste facilities, but the use of biobeds is one example where disposal may still be allowed on-farm. The siting and type of biobed are important so advice is needed to meet the new regulations.

Efforts are being made to persuade the manufacturers of sprayers to examine their designs so that the amount of liquid remaining in the sprayer, the pump and associated hoses is kept to a minimum. However, some parts of the sprayer, including the inaccessible areas of the pump, will inevitably contain pesticide deposits, and consequently those who maintain the equipment will need to be careful when dismantling the appropriate parts of sprayers.

This chapter has shown that with the correct choice of pesticide, packaging and equipment, together with the use of appropriate protective equipment, operators can apply pesticides safely with minimal exposure to the chemicals used.

References

Anon (1999a) *Dermal Exposure to Non-agricultural Pesticides: Exposure assessment document*. Health and Safety Executive.

Anon (1999b) *Risk Assessment to Risk Management: Dealing with uncertainty.* Risk Assessment and Toxicology Steering Committee, Institute for Environment and Health, Leicester.

Anon (2002) *Dermal Exposure Resulting from Liquid Contamination.* HSE/DSTL Report A-2248.

Anon (2004) *Guidelines for Good Exposure Assessment Practice for Human Health Effects of Chemicals.* IGHRC Cr 10. Institute of Environmental Health, University of Leicester.

Anon (2005) *Cholinesterase Monitoring of Pesticide Handlers in Agriculture. Report to the Legislature as required by RCW 49.17.288.* Washington State, USA.

Basford, W.D., Rose, S.C. and Carter, A.D. (2004) On-farm bioremediation (biobed) systems to limit point source pesticide pollution from sprayer mixing and wash-down areas. *Aspects of Applied Biology* **71**, 27–34.

Bjugstad, N. and Torgrimsen, T. (1996) Operator safety and plant deposits when using pesticides in greenhouses. *Journal of Agricultural Engineering Research* **65**, 205–212.

Buchanan, D., Pilkington, A., Sewell, C., Tannahill, S.N., Kidd, M.W., Cherrie, B. and Hurley, J.F. (2001) Estimation of cumulative exposure to organophosphate sheep dips in a study of chronic neurological heath effects among United Kingdom sheep dippers. *Occupational and Environmental Medicine* **58**, 694–701.

Chester, G. (1993) Evaluation of agricultural worker exposure to, and absorption of, pesticides. *Annals of Occupational Hygiene* **37**, 509–523.

Chester, G. (1995) Revised guidance document for the conduct of field studies of exposure to pesticides in use. In: P.B. Curry *et al.* (eds.), *Methods of Pesticide Exposure Assessment.* NATO Challenges of Modern Society, Plenum Press, New York, London, Vol. 19, pp. 179–215.

Chester, G. and Ward, R.J. (1983) An accurate method for measuring potential dermal exposure to pesticides. *Human Toxicology* **2**, 555–556.

Cinalli, C., Carter, D., Clark, A. and Dixon, D. (1992) *A Laboratory Method to Determine the Retention of Liquids on the Surface of Hands.* US EPA Report 747-R-92–003.

Clay, M.M. and Clarke, S.W. (1987) Effect of nebulised aerosol size on lung deposition in patients with mild asthma. *Thorax* **42**, 190–194.

Coffman, C.W., Obendorf, S.K. and Derksen, R.C. (1999) Pesticide deposition on coveralls during vineyard applications. *Archives of Environmental Contamination and Toxicology* **37**, 273–279.

Craig, I. and Mbevi, C. (1993) Contamination in the tropics. *Pesticide News* **19**, 3–5.

Curry, P.B., Iyengar, S., Maloney, P.A. and Maroni, M. (eds.) (1995), *Methods of Pesticide Exposure Assessment.* NATO/Challenges of Modern Society, Plenum Press, New York, Vol. 19, pp. 1–224.

Denovan, L.A., Lu, C., Hines, C.J. and Fenske, R.A. (2000) Saliva biomonitoring of atrazine exposure among herbicide applicators. *International Archives of Occupational and Environmental Health* **73**, 457–462.

De Vreede, J.A.F., Brouwer, D.H., Stevenson, H. and van Hemmen, J.J. (1998) Exposure and risk estimation for pesticides in high-volume spraying. *Annals of Occupational Hygiene* **42**, 151–157.

Durham, W.F. and Wolfe, H.R. (1962) Measurement of the exposure of workers to pesticides. *Bulletin of the World Health Organization* **26**, 75–91.

Fenske, R.A. (1990) Non-uniform dermal deposition patterns during occupational exposure to pesticides. *Archives of Environmental Contamination and Toxicology* **19**, 332–337.

Fenske, R.A. and Day, E.W. (2005) Assessment of exposure for pesticide handlers in agricultural, residential and institutional environments. In: Franklin, C.A. and

Worgan, J.P. (eds.), *Occupational and Residential Exposure Assessment for Pesticides*. Wiley, Chichester, pp. 13–43.

Fernando, H.E. (1956) A new design of sprayer for reducing insecticide hazards in treating rice crop. *FAO Plant Protection Bulletin* **4** 117–120.

Fogg, P. and Carter, A.D. (1998) Biobeds: The development and evaluation of a biological system for pesticide waste and washings. *BCPC Symposium* **70**, 49–58.

Fogg, P., Boxall, A.B.A., Walker, A. and Jukes, A.A. (2003a) Pesticide degradation in a 'biobed' composting substrate. *Pest Management Science* **59**, 527–537.

Fogg, P., Boxall, A.B.A., Walker, A. and Jukes, A. (2003b) Degradation and leaching potential of pesticides in biobed systems. *Pest Management Science* **60**, 645–654.

Garfitt, S.J., Jones, K., Mason, H.J. and Cocker, J. (2002) Oral and dermal exposure to propetamphos: A human volunteer study. *Toxicology Letters* **134**, 115–118.

Garthwaite, D. (2002) *A Survey of Current Farm Practices in the UK*. Report for the Crop Protection Association. Central Science Laboratory.

Gilbert, A.J. (1995) Analysis of exposure to pesticides applied in a regulated environment. In: Best, G.A. and Ruthven, A.D. (eds.), *Pesticides – Developments, Impacts, and Controls*. Royal Society of Chemistry.

Gilbert, A.J. and Bell, G.J. (1990) Test methods and criteria for selection of types of coveralls suitable for certain operations involving handling or applying pesticides. *Journal of Occupational Accidents* **11**, 255–268.

Glass, C.R., Cohen Gomez, E., Delgado Cobos, P. and Mathers, J.J. (1998) Modified spray test for protective clothing used in southern Europe. *Proceedings of 9th International Congress Pesticide Chemistry, The Food-Environment Challenge*, Westminster, London, UK. 2–7 August 1998.

Glass, C.R., Gilbert, A.J., Mathers, J.J., Martinez Vidal, J.L., Gonzalez, F.J.E., Moreira, J.F. Machera, K., Kapetanakis, E. and Capri, E. (2000) Worker exposure to pesticides – a pan European approach. *Aspects of Applied Biology* **57**, 363 –369.

Glass, C.R., Gilbert, A.J., Mathers, J.J., Lewis, R.J., Harrington, P.M. and Perez Duran, S. (2002a) Potential for operator and environmental contamination during concentrate handling in UK agriculture. *Aspects of Applied Biology* **66**, 379–386.

Glass, C.R., Gilbert, A.J., Mathers, J.J., Martinez Vidal, J.L., Egea Gonzalez, F.J., Gonzales Pradas, E., Urena Amate, D., Fernandez Perez, M., Flores Cespedes, F., Delgado Cobos, P., Cohen Gomez, E., Moreira, J.F., Santos, J., Meuling, W., Kapetanakis, E., Goumenaki, E., Papaeliakis, M., Machera, K., Goumenou, M.P., Capri, E., Trevisan, M., Wilkins, R.M., Garratt, J.A., Tuomainen, A. and Kangas, J. (2002b) *The Assessment of Operator, Bystander and Environmental Exposure to Pesticides*. Final Report EUR_20489 Project contract SMT4-CT96–2048.

Glass, C.R., Mathers, J.J., Lewis, R.J., Harrington, P.M., Gilbert, A.J. and Smith, S. (2004) Understanding exposure to agricultural pesticide concentrates. Report to HSE unpublished.

Gustin, C.A., Moran, S.J., Fuhrman, J.D., Kurtzweil, M.L., Kronenberg, J.M., Gustafson, D.I. and Marshall, M.A. (2005) Applicator exposure to acetochlor based on biomonitoring. *Regulatory Toxicology and Pharmacology* **43**, 141–149.

Hall, R.M., Heitbrink, W.A. and Reed, L.D. (2002) Evaluation of a cab using real-time aerosol counting instrumentation. *Applied Occupational and Environmental Hygiene* **17**, 46–54.

Hamey, P.Y. (2001) The need for appropriate use information to refine pesticide user exposure assessments. *Annals of Occupational Hygiene* **45**, S69–S79.

Harrington, P., Mathers, J., Lewis, R., Perez Duran, S. and Glass, R. (2005) Potential exposure to pesticides during amateur applications of home and garden products. In: Lichtfouse, E., Schwarzbauer, J. and Robert, D. (eds.), *Environmental Chemistry; Green Chemistry and Pollutants in Ecosystems* **26**, 530–537.

Harris, D.A., Johnson, K.S. and Ogilvy, J.M.E. (1991) A system for the treatment of waste water from agrochemical production and field use. *Brighton Crop Protection Conference – Weeds* 715–722.

Henriksen, V.V., Helweg, A., Spliid, N.H., Felding, G. and Stenvang, L. (2003) Capacity of model biobeds to retain and degrade mecoprop and isoproturon. *Pest Management Science* **59**, 1076–1082.

HSE (2002) *Dermal Exposure Resulting from Liquid Contamination*. HSE Books, Sudbury.

Hughes, E., Zalts, A., Ojeda, J., Montserrat, J. and Glass, R. (2004) Potential pesticide exposure of small-scale vegetable growers in Moreno district. *Aspects of Applied Biology* **71**, 399–404.

Krieger, R.I. (1995) Pesticide exposure assessment. *Toxicology Letters* **82**, 65–72.

Krieger, R.I. and Dinoff, T.M. (2000) Malathion deposition, metabolite clearance, and cholinesterase status of date dusters and harvesters in California. *Archives of Environmental Contamination and Toxicology* **38**, 546–553.

Krieger, R.I., Bernard, C.E., Dinoff, T.M., Ross, J.H. and Williams, R.L. (2001) Biomonitoring of persons exposed to insecticides used in residences. *Annals of Occupational Hygiene* **45**, S143–S153.

Kummer, R. and van Sittert, N.J. (1986) Field studies on health effects from the application of two organophosphorus insecticide formulations by hand-held ULV to cotton. *Toxicology Letters* **33**, 7–24.

Landers, A. (2004) Protecting the operator – are we making an impact? *Aspects of Applied Biology* **71**, 357–364.

Llewellyn, D.M., Brazier, A., Brown, R., Cocker, J., Evans, M.L., Hampton, J., Nutley, B.P. and White, J. (1996) Occupational exposure to permethrin during its use as a public hygiene insecticide. *Annals of Occupational Hygiene* **40**, 499–509.

Lock, E.A. and Wilks, M.F. (2001) Paraquat. In: Krieger, R.I. (ed.), *Handbook of Pesticide Toxicology*, 2nd edn. Academic Press, San Diego, pp. 1559–1603.

Machado-Neto, J.G., Matuo, T. and Matuo, Y.K. (1998) Efficiency of safety measures applied to a manual knapsack sprayer for paraquat application to maize (*Zea mays* L.) *Archives of Environmental Contamination and Toxicology* **35**, 69–701.

Machera, K., Goumenou, M., Kapetanakis, E., Kalamarakis, A. and Glass, R. (2001) Determination of potential dermal and inhalation exposure of operators, following spray applications of the fungicide penconazole in vineyards and greenhouses. *Fresenius Environmental Bulletin* **10**, 464–469.

Machera, K., Kapetanakis, E., Charistou, A., Goumenaki, E. and Glass, R. (2002) Evaluation of potential dermal exposure of pesticide spray operators in greenhouses by use of visual tracers. *Journal of Environmental Science and Health* **37**, 113–121.

Marin Juan, A., Martinez-Vidal, J.L., Egea Gonzalez, F.J., Garrido Frenich, A., Belomonte Vega, A., Glass, C.R. and Sykes, M. (2004) Biological monitoring of greenhouse workers in Almeria. *Aspects of Applied Biology* **71**, 405–408.

Matthews, G.A (2001) Dermal exposure of hands to pesticides. In: Maibach, I. (ed.), *Toxicology of Skin*. Taylor and Francis, pp. 179–182.

Maumbe, B.M. and Swinton, S.M. (2003) Hidden health costs of pesticide use in Zimbabwe's smallholder cotton growers. *Social Science and Medicine* **57**, 1559–1571.

Mekonnen, Y. and Agonafir, T. (2002) Pesticide sprayers' knowledge, attitude and practice of pesticide use on agricultural farms of Ethiopia. *Occupational Medicine* **52**, 311–315.

Meuling, W.J.A., Franssen, A.C., Brouwer, D.H. and van Hemmen, J.J. (1997) The influence of skin moisture on the dermal absorption of propoxur in human volunteers: Consideration for biological monitoring practices. *The Science of the Total Environment* **199**, 165–172.

Moreira, J.F., Santos, J. and Glass, C.R. (1999) Personal protective equipment penetration during application of plant protection products. XIVth International Plant Protection Congress, Jerusalem, Israel, July 25–30.

Nelson, C., Laughlin, J., Kim, C., Rigakis, K., Mastura, R. and Scholten, L. (1992) Laundering as decontamination of apparel fabrics: Residues of pesticides from six chemical classes. *Archives of Environmental Contamination and Toxicology* **23**. 85–90.

Ngowi, A.V.F., Maeda, D.N. and Partanen, T.J. (2001a) Assessment of the ability of health care providers to treat and prevent adverse health effects of pesticides in agricultural areas of Tanzania. *International Journal of Occupational Medicine and Environmental Health* **14**, 349–356.

Ngowi, A.V.F., Maeda, D.N., Partanen, T.J., Sanga, M.P. and Mbise, G. (2001b) Acute health effects of organophosphorus pesticides in Tanzanian small-scale coffee growers. *Journal of Exposure Analysis and Environmental Epidemiology* **11**, 335–339.

Nutley, B.P., Berry, H.F., Roff, M., Brown, R.H., Niven, K.J.M. and Robertson, A. (1995) The assessment of operator risk from sheep dipping operations using organophosphate based dips. In: Best, G. and Ruthven, D. (eds.), *Pesticides – Developments, Impacts and Controls*. Royal Society of Chemistry, London, pp. 43–53.

Nuyttens, D., Windey, S., Braekman, P., de Moor, A. and Sonck, B. (2004) Comparison of operator exposure for five different greenhouse spraying applications. *Aspects of Applied Biology* **71**, 349–356.

Ohayo-Mitoko, G.J.A., Kromhout, H. Karumba, P.N. and Boleij, J.S.M. (1999) Identification of determinants of pesticide exposure among Kenyan Agricultural workers using empirical modelling. *Annals of Occupational Hygiene* **43**, 519–525.

Ramwell, C.T., Johnson, P.D., Boxall, A.B.A. and Rimmer, D.A. (2004) Pesticide residues on the external surfaces of field-crop sprayers: Environmental impact. *Pest Management Science* **60**, 795–802.

Renwick, A.G. (1991) Safety factors and establishment of acceptable daily intake. *Food Additives and Contaminants* **8**, 135–150.

Roff, M.W. (1994) A novel lighting system for the measurement of dermal exposure using a fluorescent dye and an image processor. *Annals of Occupational Hygiene* **38**, 903–919.

Ross, J.H., Driver, J.H., Cochran, R.C., Thongsinthusak, T. and Krieger, R.I. (2001) Could pesticide toxicology studies be more relevant to occupational risk assessment? *Annals of Occupational Hygiene* **1001**, S5–S17.

Shaw, A., Lin, Y.J. and Pfell, E. (1996) Effect of abrasion on protective properties of polyester and cotton/polyester blend fabrics. *Bulletin of Environmental Contamination and Toxicology* **56**, 935–941.

Shaw, A., Lin, Y.J. and Pfell, E. (1997) Qualitative and quantitative analysis of diazinon in fabric exposed to various simulated sunlight and humidity conditions. *Bulletin of Environmental Contamination and Toxicology* **59**, 389–395.

Shaw, A., Nomula, R. and Patel, B. (2000) Protective clothing and application controls for pesticide application in India: A field study. In: Nelson, C.N. and Henry, N.W. (eds.), *Performance of Protective Clothing: Issues and priorities for the 21st century*. Seventh Volume, ASTM STP 1386.

Sutherland, J.A., King, W.J., Dobson, H.M. Ingram, W.R., Attique, M.R. and Sanjrani, W. (1990) Effect of application volume and method on spray operator contamination by insecticide during cotton spraying. *Crop Protection* **9**, 343–350.

Thornhill, E.W., Matthews, G.A. and Clayton, J.S. (1996) Potential operator exposure to insecticides: A comparison between knapsack and CDA spinning disc sprayers. *Proceedings, Brighton Conference* **3**, 1175–1180.

Tunstall, J.P. and Matthews, G.A. (1965) Contamination hazards in using knapsack sprayers. *Empire Cotton Growing Review* **42**(3), 193–196.

Van Drooge, H.L., Groeneveld, C.N. and Schipper, H.J. (2001) Data on application frequency of pesticide for risk assessment purposes. *Annals of Occupational Hygiene* **45**, S95–S101.

Van Hemmen, J.J. and Brouwer, D.H. (1997) Exposure assessment for pesticides: Operators and harvesters risk evaluation and risk management. *Med. Fac. Landbouww. University of Gent* **62/2**, 113–130.

Van Hemmen, J.J. and van der Jagt, K.E. (2005) Generic operator exposure databases. In: Franklin, C.A. and Worgan, J.P. (eds.), *Occupational and Residential Exposure Assessment for Pesticides*. Wiley, Chichester, pp. 173–208.

Wester, R.C. and Maibach, H.I. (1985) *In vivo* percutaneous absorption and decontamination of pesticides in humans. *Journal of Toxicology and Environmental Health* **16**, 25–37.

Wester, R.C., Sedik, L., Melenderes, J., Logan, F., Maibach, H.I. and Russel, I. (1993) Percutaneous absorption of diazinon in humans. *Food and Chemical Toxicology* **31**, 569–572.

Wicke, H., Backer, G. and Frieβleben, R. (1999) Comparison of spray operator exposure during orchard spraying with hand-held equipment fitted with standard and air injector nozzles. *Crop Protection* **18**, 509–516.

Wolf, T.M., Gallender, K.S., Downer, R.A., Hall, F.R., Fraley, F.W. and Pompeo, M.P. (1999) Contribution of aerosols generated during mixing and loading of pesticides to operator inhalation exposure. *Toxicology Letters* **105**, 31–38.

Wolfe, H.R. (1976) Field exposure to airborne particles. In: Lee, R.E. (ed.), *Air Pollution from Pesticides*. CRC Press, Cleveland, pp. 137–161.

Advice for farmers on protection when applying pesticides is available in a BCPC booklet *Safety Equipment Handbook*.

5 Spray drift, bystander, resident and worker exposure

This chapter considers the movement of spray droplets and pesticide deposits from treated fields, and the effects on bystanders and people living near agricultural areas. The exposure of those working in crops that have been sprayed, namely farm workers, who come into contact with the pesticide deposits is also considered.

The movement of spray droplets by the wind at the time of a spray application to areas that are outside the treated fields can cause unacceptable effects depending on the type of pesticide. Insecticides may adversely affect bees and other beneficial or non-target insects, while herbicides can affect vegetation, which can in turn cause a reduction in non-target species by effects on habitats and food sources. The subject of spray drift has become a very emotive issue as the general public have felt that airborne spray is the cause of many illnesses. In the UK, any specific complaint made by a member of the public, related to agricultural use of pesticides, excluding sheep treatments covered by the Medicines Act 1968, is examined carefully by the Pesticide Incident Appraisal Panel (PIAP), which is administered by the HSE. In 2003–4 there were 204 complaints, of which 62 involved allegations of ill-health. The other 142 complaints were mostly related to environmental concerns. There were eight convictions during the year to enforce the regulations (Anon, 2004). Only in a small proportion of the incidents reported is a definite occurrence of spray drift confirmed as a possible cause of the complaint. In many cases the complaint follows detection of the odour of the active ingredient of the pesticide, and also in some cases the solvent or carrier used in the formulation, due more to vapour drift rather than to the movement of spray droplets. This is because of the sensitivity of the human nose to certain odours at extremely low concentrations. The system of reporting to HSE has been criticised as it deals almost entirely with acute symptoms, and very few cases of chronic illness are reported; typically, complaints take weeks or months to be investigated. Public sensitivity to spray drift has increased, especially where new housing developments are situated close to agricultural areas. The Royal Commission, recognising criticism of the PIAP, has recommended that the role of monitoring bystander exposure should be part of the Health Protection Agency under the Department of Health rather than the HSE.

Downwind drift of vapour may also occur after a spray application from foliar deposits due to the volatility of the pesticide, if temperatures are sufficiently high. Widespread serious phytotoxic effects on some broad-leaved vegetable crops occurred during the 1970s in England, when there was exceptionally warm weather after a volatile herbicide had been applied on cereals (Elliot and Wilson, 1983). This led to improvements in the formulation of the herbicide to reduce volatility. In Canada, drift potential of the butyl ester was eight- to ten-fold greater than that from the dimethylamine formulation of 2,4-D in trials where 25–30% of the butyl ester formulation was collected as vapour drift in the half-hour after spraying (Grover *et al.*, 1972). Vapour drift can occur more than 12 hours after application, especially if temperatures are high.

What is drift?

Himel (1974) defined spray drift into two categories, namely exo- and endo-drift (Fig. 5.1).

Exo-drift

This is the movement of spray droplets beyond the edge of a treated field. Most recent studies have been concerned with the deposition of spray droplets on the ground or other horizontal surfaces over a relatively short distance

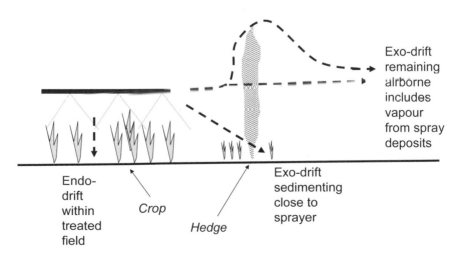

Fig. 5.1 Exo- and endo-drift.

downwind of a field. A much smaller proportion of an agricultural spray made up of the smallest droplets will tend to remain airborne, and these droplets can travel over very long distances if the meteorological conditions favour their movement.

Endo-drift

This is the distribution of a pesticide within a field, but not on the intended target. Thus, some of a foliar spray may fail to be deposited on leaves and sediment on the ground. Subsequent movement of this pesticide deposit by leaching through the soil profile can lead to contamination of groundwater, if the pesticide molecule is sufficiently mobile in soil and not adsorbed onto the soil particles. This endo-drift could also become exo-drift, if heavy rain or irrigation washed the soil surface deposit into the nearest ditch or waterway. Although not spray drift in the strict sense of downwind movement of droplets, another source of pesticide contamination of surface water or drains is the water used to wash a sprayer or if there is any spillage from a pesticide container.

Peak levels of pesticide in river water samples, caused by surface run-off following storms involving 6.8–18.4 mm rain/day, were from 2 to 41 times higher than the levels recorded due to spray drift (0.04–0.07 µg/l), even when the river discharge rate was much greater at 7–22.4 m³/s instead of 0.28 m³/s (Schulz, 2001). In Germany, 24 g of pesticides was found in each farmyard run-off during the application period, presumably caused by cleaning the spraying equipment (Neumann *et al.*, 2002). This has led to the need for an additional water tank on the sprayer so at least the inside of the tank is washed in the field and the washings are used to spray the last part of a field.

How is drift measured?

An international standard for measurement of drift (ISO 22866) is designed to cover both short-range downwind sedimentation of spray and longer range airborne drift of the smaller spray droplets.

Droplets that sediment

Most attention has been given to the spray that is collected at ground level (Fig. 5.2). Trials have been concerned with the distribution of spray obtained with different types of equipment, but for registration requirements the sedimentation data have been needed in risk assessments of drift on to surface water, and this has led to the adoption of buffer zones. The trajectory of droplets larger than 200 µm from a tractor boom is influenced primarily

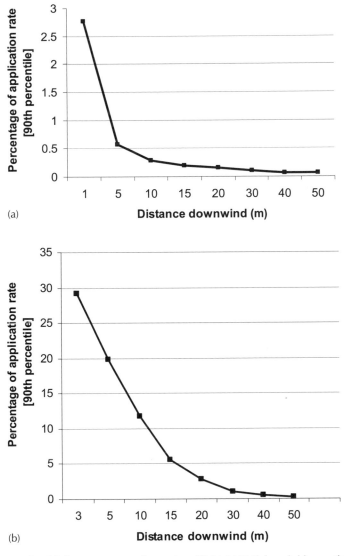

Fig. 5.2 Example of drift measurements from edge of field. (a) Drift from field crop. (b) Drift from orchard early season.

by gravity, so fall out on a horizontal surface occurs mostly within about 5 m from the end of the boom, hence this basic distance is used for buffer zones to protect water-courses.

Different sampling methods have been used, but most have relied on sampling spray deposited on a horizontal surface. Measurements have been made when applying pesticides that are easily measured, but most assessments are made with a tracer dye quantified by spectrofluorometric analysis. The dye used should be non-toxic and relatively inexpensive. The food colourant tartrazine is one dye that has been used. A dye also must be photo-stable as the samples cannot all be collected simultaneously. Some drift studies have used EDTA chelates of metals as spray tracers, as this allows spraying with different equipment over the same target area to be carried out and the deposits of each tracer on the same samples to be separated (Cross *et al.*, 2001). Neutron activation analysis, using dysposium chloride added to the spray, has also been used to detect drift (Dobson *et al.*, 1983). A combination of a fluorescent dye and pesticide is sometimes used to allow a large number of samples to be examined qualitatively, thereby restricting chemical analyses to subsamples that relate to different levels of spray coverage (Matthews and Johnstone, 1968).

Glass surfaces have the advantage that when measuring a pesticide or tracer, the deposit can be easily washed off and measured quantitatively. Petri dishes have been used but these suffer from a raised edge that can affect the air-flow and thus movement of smaller droplets close to the dish. Flat glass plates avoid this problem, but they must be kept exactly horizontal during sampling, as deposition can be influenced even if the plates are placed at a slight angle. In studying the distribution of spray across the swath of an aircraft, Johnstone and Matthews (1965) used table tennis balls mounted on pins to sample the spray (which contained a red dye tracer) to avoid the difficulty of having plates set correctly in a grass field.

The amount of spray deposited will decline as distances downwind increase; thus, the sample size must be sufficiently large to collect a measurable amount of the tracer. An individual sample of 100 cm^2 is usually considered necessary. The ISO standard for drift measurement also requires a minimum total area of 1000 cm^2 to be sampled. Apart from having samples at different distances downwind, ideally the sampling line is replicated to allow for variations in wind speed and direction while taking the sample. Often, costs prevent adequate numbers of samples being taken. Visual assessments of spray drift, at least over short distances, can be made by setting out small strips of water-sensitive paper that change colour when water droplets are deposited on them.

The cost of performing field assessments of spray drift and variability due to changes in wind velocity and direction have led to efforts to assess the potential spray drift from different nozzles in a wind tunnel (Fig. 5.3).

Airborne droplets

Droplets that remain airborne are generally smaller than 100 µm in size, and unless the liquid is non-volatile they will become smaller in flight. Efficient sampling of these small droplets is more difficult as they can bypass a solid object in their path, when carried in the airflow. Passive samplers, such as a suspended 2-mm diameter polythene line, have acceptable collection effi-

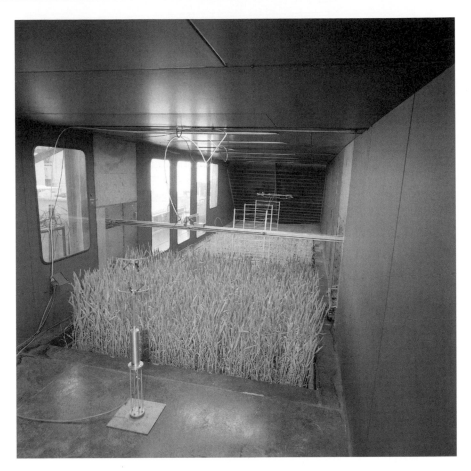

Fig. 5.3 Measuring potential drift under wind-tunnel conditions (Silsoe Research Institute).

ciency, and dye can be recovered and quantified at reasonable cost (Gilbert and Bell, 1988; Miller, 1993) (Fig. 5.4).

These lines are less expensive to use than samplers that draw air through a filter at a calibrated rate. However, washing the filter allows the amount of tracer to be quantified in relation to the volume of air sampled and the sampling time. Small units can be attached to a person in order to sample air near the face (breathing zone) for assessing the inhalation risk of a pesticide. A cascade impactor is a specialised high-volume air sampler that separates samples in relation to the size of droplets. Pumps to draw air through the sampler require a source of power, so field samples are often taken with rotary samplers, such as rotorods, which can be battery-operated.

Lidar measurements have been made to assess long-range drift to validate models such as the USDA Forest Service Cramer-Barry-Grim (FSCBG). Stoughton *et al.* (1997) reported that aerial sprays over a forest canopy drifted

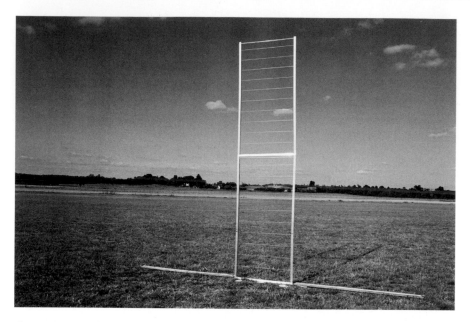

Fig. 5.4   Sampler for airborne drift of spray droplets (Silsoe Research Institute).

more than 2000 m from the spray line, which was further than predicted during near-neutral conditions.

Briand *et al.* (2002) compared different samplers, in conjunction with gas chromatography-mass spectrometry, to evaluate spray drift from an orchard. Compared to earlier studies, the relatively high concentrations that were detected in the gas phase indicated that evaporation in the high temperatures from small droplets allowed them to drift. Thus, temperature and relative humidity as well as the physical properties of the pesticide will influence the vapour and particle distribution, making it important to differentiate between drift and post-application transfer from deposits.

In Germany, the time-weighted air concentration of pesticides downwind of a barley field due to spray drift was highest during the first 2 hours after application, and then decreased. Over 21 hours, up to 0.58 $\mu g/m^3$ was detected at 10 m downwind. Volatile insecticides were detected at up to 200 m in the first 2 hours, but this was below the limit of quantification (Siebers *et al.*, 2003).

Few studies have sampled air in the UK for pesticides, but where these have been done (Turnbull, 1995) the highest quantities observed over 24 or 48 hours were in samples taken near to field applications. One sample was just over 2000 pg/m^3, which is 42,000 times less than the air concentration measured at the bystander position 8 m from the boom. Mean values of pesticides in air were generally less than 400 pg/m^3. Similar air quality studies elsewhere have generally detected the most volatile of pesticides, such as methyl bromide, which is used to fumigate soil (Lee *et al.*, 2002).

The amount of a pesticide in the air declines due to dilution with other air, removal by rain, and degradation of the pesticide. Restricting the use of organochlorine insecticides has led to a 10-fold decrease in gamma HCH (lindane) deposits in the atmosphere in France (Teil *et al.*, 2004). In contrast, air samples in Birmingham showed no decline in gamma HCH, but DDT concentrations were much lower in 1999–2000 compared to 1997–98 (Harrad and Mao, 2004).

Rainfall will wash airborne spray droplets from the atmosphere. In a study in Iowa, concentrations of herbicides detected in rain varied from non-detectable amounts to as much as 154 µg/l, the latter occurring when atrazine had been applied on an extremely humid day immediately followed by <10 mm rain. This only occurred locally, however, with other collectors detecting 1.7 µg/l. Total annual samples in rain represented less than 0.1% of the amount applied (Hatfield *et al.*, 1996). Similar data from Germany confirms that atrazine was detected in rain (Epple *et al.*, 2002). Other data relating to amounts of pesticide in rainwater (which are generally below µg/l levels) were noted by Unsworth *et al.* (1999), who reported the long-range transport of pesticides in the atmosphere to the IUPAC Commission on Agrochemicals and the Environment.

Bystander exposure

A bystander is a person who is located within, or adjacent to, an area where pesticides are being applied or have just been applied, but whose presence is quite incidental and unrelated to the application of the pesticide. There is a risk that some of the spray drifting downwind could be deposited on their body, especially if no action is taken to avoid exposure (Fig. 5.5). A bystander who happens to be walking near a field while it is being sprayed would not be wearing any personal protective clothing (PPE). Workers who enter a field, for example, to harvest a crop, are considered separately below. However, in addition to people walking near fields that are being sprayed, concern has been expressed about spray drifting across field boundaries into adjacent gardens and houses, occupied by 'residential neighbours'.

An assessment of exposure to bystanders is required under the proposed conditions of use prior to authorisation of plant protection products under the European Directive 91/414 EEC. In the UK, exposure of bystanders to spray was studied by Gilbert and Bell (1988), who used tracer studies to measure the amount of airborne tracer that reached the breathing zone, as well as the spray deposited on the clothing and uncovered skin of a person standing 8 m downwind from the edge of an area treated with a tractor sprayer with a horizontal boom. In these trials, hydraulic nozzles applied 300 l/ha of a dye that was extracted from the whole disposable overall. The exposure was expressed as ml from the total surface (2 m²) per upwind pass

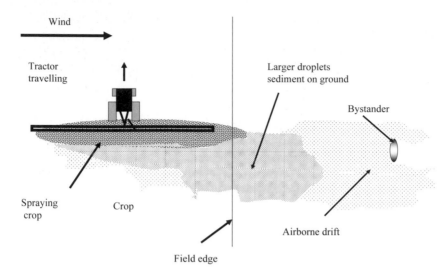

Fig. 5.5 Diagram to show position of sampling for bystander exposure.

of the sprayer. Twenty layers of nylon gauze were used in a respirator to collect spray reaching the breathing zone.

Several trials were carried out so that differences in wind speed were taken into account in estimating potential exposure of the bystander under a range of weather conditions. On average, a bystander was exposed to 0.1 ml of spray for a single pass of the sprayer. A three-fold increase in the total deposition on a bystander, who stayed in the same position, was estimated to account for any spray that may reach the bystander as the sprayer moved further away upwind. However, more of the spray would be deposited on the crop, especially as the smallest airborne droplets tend to be carried around a solid body. The trials confirmed that relatively few droplets will remain close enough to the breathing zone to be inhaled. The amount of spray collected on the gauze filter in the breathing zone indicated a mean potential inhalation exposure of 0.02 ml/m^3. This is translated into an inhalation exposure of 0.006 ml spray, assuming an exposure period of 5 minutes, a respiratory rate of $3.6 \text{ m}^3/\text{h}$, and that all of the pesticide was absorbed. Inevitably, under field conditions with variations in wind speed and direction, there will be some variability in measurements. The adoption of a mean value has been criticised with the suggestion that more account should be taken of the probability of more exposure under some conditions.

The distance of 8 m was chosen as any person closer would be more likely to have some involvement in the pesticide application, and therefore be wearing at least overalls. However, more recent experiments (Figs. 5.6 and 5.7) have assessed exposure of a bystander at 1 and 5 m from a 12-m

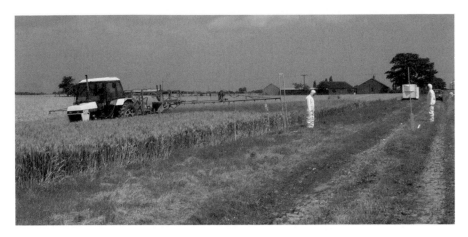

Fig. 5.6 Using a coloured dye to measure exposure to bystanders at two distances downwind of the end of the spray boom (photograph CSL).

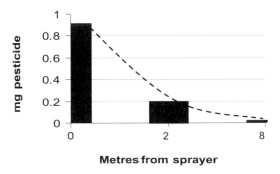

Metres from sprayer

Fig. 5.7 Decrease in exposure at different distances downwind of the boom.

boom sprayer, fitted with 110° standard fan nozzles, treating a wheat crop (DEFRA, 2003). Potential dermal exposure at 1 m compared to 5 m downwind increased seven-fold at low wind speeds (about 1.5 m/s), but there was a less than a two-fold increase at the highest wind speed (5.1 m/s). Overall exposure was similar to the maximum values obtained by Gilbert and Bell (1988). When air-induction nozzles, producing a coarser spray (Piggott and Matthews, 1999) were used, bystander exposure was reduced. Spray drifting beyond the edge of a crop can be reduced by other application techniques, including the use of a downward-directed air-assisted spray and operating nozzles at a lower pressure.

In a separate study of orchard spraying, the bystander at 8 m downwind was exposed to 3.7 ml of spray with 0.002 ml/person in the breathing zone (Lloyd *et al.*, 1987). The increased exposure is related to the spray being directed up into trees, so more droplets are airborne compared to the arable situation with downwardly directed sprays.

Bystander exposure is therefore directly related to the proportion of droplets in a spray that remain airborne.

For the bystander, the larger droplets still airborne may impact on parts of the body, but the smallest will tend to be carried in the air-flow around the body. Droplets in the size range that can be inhaled (<10 μm) are those most likely to be carried by wind away from a bystander. Clearly, the coarser the spray, the less the exposure to the bystander, as confirmed when air-induction nozzles (which produce only a small volume of spray in droplets below 100 μm diameter, typically <5%) were used.

Generally, in open fields inhalation exposure is negligible due to the extremely small volume of spray in droplets small enough to be inhaled into the lungs. Nevertheless, there is concern about downwind spray drift, which may be deposited on bystanders, as this is the cause of some reports to the HSE. However, tests have shown that, in general, the exposure of unprotected bystanders is only a fraction compared with the spray operator (Gilbert and Bell, 1988). In practice, people entering fields after a pesticide treatment may be aware of an odour, which may be due to the pesticide or to a volatile chemical used in the formulation. Exposure to the deposits, once they have dried, will depend on how dislodgeable the spray deposit is when the bystander is in contact with it. There is also a risk of vapour from spray deposits, which is likely to be highest immediately after an application.

In a study in Washington, USA, high-volume air samplers were used to detect the organophosphate (OP) insecticide methamidophos applied by aircraft to five fields of potato crops located around a residential community. Data from samples taken 12 hours before, during, and 24 hours after the application were compared with a predictive model, which tended to underestimate immediately after the spray but to overestimate the emission the next day (Ramaprasad *et al.*, 2004). Nevertheless, the data demonstrated the potentially high risk of inhalation exposure after the spraying was completed, when a volatile pesticide has been aerially applied. The importance of pesticide volatility was stressed by Scheyer *et al.* (2005), who showed that in an urban environment insecticides such as gamma HCH can be detected at between 0.01 and 1 ng/m^3 following soil–air transfer, and that in 2003 endosulfan was also present during the summer months in eastern France. Recently in California, agrochemical companies have been requested for more information on 787 pesticide products to assess their volatile organic content (VOC). This is to meet Federal Clean Air Standards for ambient air quality, the aim being to keep the VOC of pesticide products capped at 20%.

Risk assessment in the UK assumes that bystanders are exposed at the same daily level for three months, which is considered to be far longer than those living next door to a treated field would actually experience.

Furthermore, the highly toxic pesticides such as methamidophos are not approved in the UK, and with changes in formulation to reduce volatility and improvements in application technology to minimise spray drift the potential for exposure to bystanders in the vicinity of treated fields has been reduced. When the Advisory Committee on Pesticides (ACP) considered exposure of residents to sprays during the cropping season from nearby fields, it concluded that the current approach was probably protective of long-term bystander exposure. While the Royal Commission on Environmental Pollution, in its report on bystander exposure, considered that the methodology described above was conservative and protective in toxicological terms, it highlighted a number of shortcomings of the approach used by the PSD to assess bystander exposure to pesticides. In particular, the approach was limited by using the mean of measurements taken on a person standing at one distance (8 m) downwind of a sprayer. As people vary in their sensitivity to chemicals (Fig. 5.8), the Royal Commission suggested that risk management urgently needed probabilistic models to take account of worst-case situations. It was also felt that people should be able to know not only what

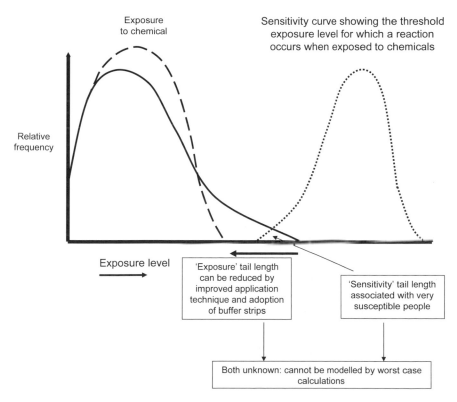

Fig. 5.8 Differences in sensitivity of individuals in relation to distribution of bystander exposure. (Adapted from an unpublished diagram by Professor Brian Hoskins, Royal Commission on Environmental Pollution.)

chemicals have been sprayed but also when they are due to be sprayed, as such information is important when examining anybody who might be ill as a result of exposure to the pesticide.

Residential exposure

Considerable concern has been raised by people living in houses close to farmland (Fig. 5.9), who have alleged ill health due to pesticides being used on neighbouring fields and drifting on to their property. However, in addition to any spray that may drift into residential properties, pesticides are now also used in homes and gardens, both in rural and urban areas. The extent to which homes are treated will vary significantly, but in warmer climates and where buildings have significant timber construction (requiring structural pest control), insecticides are applied for vectors of disease, particularly mosquitoes and flies, for household pests such as cockroaches, termites and ants, and for other pests. Garden use most often relates to herbicides used on lawns, though fungicides and insecticides are also used to protect flowers and some vegetables. It has been estimated that 90% of all US households use pesticides (Driver and Whitmyre, 1996). In the UK, only a limited number of pesticides are registered for non-professional use, and some of these are now marketed primarily in ready-to-use formulations packed in trigger-operated hand-sprayers or pressure-packs. As in many countries, these products are readily available in garden centres and supermarkets.

In the UK, there is little information available about how household pesticides are used. In one study involving a sample of 147 parents, despite safety being an important issue, one-third said they would not follow the label instructions exactly and almost 50% considered the labels to be inadequate and difficult to understand (Grey *et al.*, 2004).

This led to very few taking notice of the warnings on the label. Although it is this type of behaviour that limits which pesticides may be permitted for domestic use, it remains a concern that instructions are poorly understood or followed. Amateur application by householders is usually only for a brief period, typically less than 10 minutes, so exposure is usually confined to the fingers when using a pressure-pack dispenser (Roff *et al.*, 1998).

Apart from potential direct exposure when using a pesticide, residents can take residues of pesticides into their houses on clothing (especially agricultural workers) and/or on shoes by walking over treated surfaces. In areas with fleas on animals, carpets and furniture, residents will also be exposed to insecticides by touching treated surfaces. This is of particular concern with children crawling on carpets and transferring residues by the hand-to-mouth exposure route.

Residue transfer from a treated surface can be assessed using whole-body dosimeters (all-cotton suits, cotton socks and cotton gloves are worn).

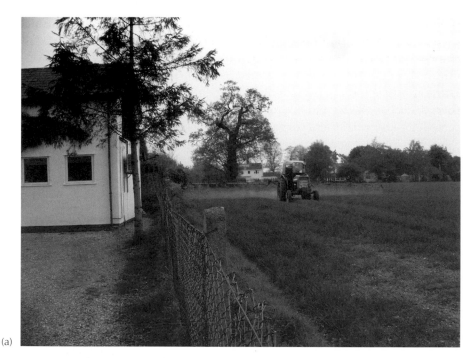

(a)

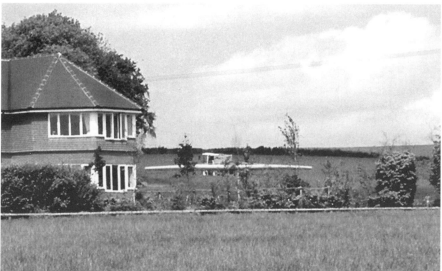

(b)

Fig. 5.9 Examples of houses close to treated field, without a garden or hedge between the house and sprayer. (a) In Norfolk (supplied by Georgina Downs, photograph by Vincent Fallon). (b) Sprayer near a house but fitted with an airsleeve to direct spray downward into the crop (photograph from Alison Craig, PAN UK).

A standardised exercise routine (referred to as Jazzercize) is followed to represent daily human activities to assess exposure by maximum contact with treated surfaces (Krieger *et al.*, 2001; Driver *et al.*, 2005). These studies can be combined with the biomonitoring of pesticides or their breakdown products detected in urine samples. In one study, 1.6 mg of the insecticide chlorpyrifos was extracted from the whole-body dosimeters, which was significantly below the amount estimated using US EPA operating procedures. Urine samples indicated that only 1.3 μg chlorpyrifos had been absorbed (Bernard *et al.*, 2001). Other studies have indicated that the human skin removes substantially less pesticide residue from treated surfaces than when a surface is wiped or a polyurethane foam roller is used to sample a surface. Hand contact averaged approximately 1–6 ng/cm^2 of chlorpyrifos-treated carpet contacted – that is, <1% of the amount deposited on the carpet 3.5 hours earlier (Lu and Fenske, 1999). Brouwer *et al.* (1999) found adherence of 1.07 μg/cm^2 after twelve contacts of a hand on a contaminated surface – that is, a transfer efficiency of ≤2%.

Sampling in a metropolitan and an agricultural area of Washington State, USA, revealed quantifiable levels of azinphos methyl and chlorpyrifos on children's hands or their toys, that suggested a greater potential exposure in agricultural families (Lu *et al.*, 2004). This contrasted with dietary studies as more samples of food for non-agricultural children had quantifiable amounts of OP pesticides. One application technique used in residences is referred to as a 'crack and crevice' treatment (Fig. 5.10). The aim is to get the insecticide into cracks in surfaces, such as brickwork, where cockroaches and other

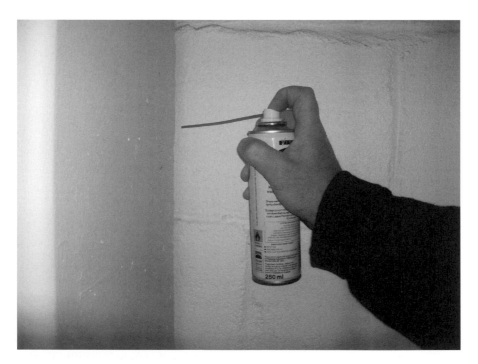

Fig. 5.10   A crack and crevice treatment with small applicator (photograph GAM).

nuisance insects may hide. In one study in the USA 1.29 g of chlorpyrifos was applied to 'harbourages' in the kitchen using 259 ml of liquid (Stout and Mason, 2003). Over a 21-day study, chlorpyrifos was dispersed into the air and distributed to other parts of the house, being detected on surgical sponge samplers (Fig. 5.11). The deposition was highest in the kitchen, but decayed over the sampling period. The data confirmed that crack and crevice treatments minimise human exposure compared to the use of pressure-packs (total release aerosols) (Mason *et al.*, 2000).

In an earlier study in California, house dust samples from eleven homes and hand-wipe samples from children in each house were analysed for 33 and 9 pesticides, respectively (Bradman *et al.*, 1997). Ten pesticides, including chlorpyrifos and diazinon, were detected in greater amounts from homes with a farm worker compared to those with no farm worker. Apart from two houses, the levels detected were below 33 ppm. The 'take home' residues of pesticides is clearly a significant factor in children's exposure to pesticides in rural areas (Garry, 2004), especially where the more toxic insecticides are used in agriculture, though the uneducated use of dispensers in a home is also a crucial source of exposure to pesticides. Lu *et al.* (2000) also reported five-fold higher concentrations of pesticide metabolites in children living in agricultural areas compared to reference children with 0.01 µg/ml.

Epidemiological studies have been conducted to determine whether there is an association between the close proximity of residences to farmland and

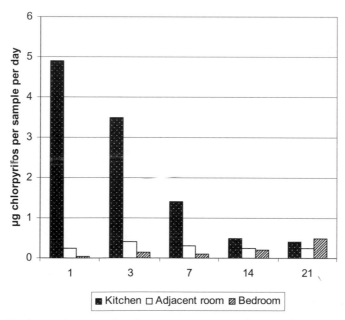

Fig. 5.11 Distribution from a crack and crevice treatment in a house in the USA (adapted from Stout, D.M. and Mason, M.A. (2003) *Atmospheric Environment* **37**, 5539–5549).

the incidence of illness. In one study in California, the incidence of breast cancer was studied among 329,000 active and retired females enrolled in the State Teachers Retirement Scheme (Reynolds *et al.*, 2004). Their analyses suggested that the incidence of breast cancer was not elevated in areas where there had been a recent high use of pesticides. In a study in two counties in the UK, spatial association between three selected pesticides and breast cancer incidence rates was found in rural Leicestershire, but not in Lincolnshire or in urban areas (Muir *et al.*, 2004). Three of the four pesticides were aldicarb (used as a granule for nematode control in potato fields), atrazine (herbicide) and lindane (used in buildings to treat timber), as these were considered to be 'oestrogenic'. The techniques used were able to rule out strong associations, but a much larger and expensive study of individuals would be required to detect a smaller risk.

Levels of organochlorine pesticides, including DDT and its metabolites, were detected in 200 women living in an area of Spain with intensive greenhouse agriculture who provided adipose tissue and blood samples during surgery. As these chemicals can be mobilised in the body during pregnancy and lactation, health consequences for the children of those exposed is of some concern, and further research is needed on infant exposure in this way (Botella *et al.*, 2004). Fortunately, as the organochlorines have been banned, except DDT for vector control, levels of these pesticides in humans are expected to decline.

In Japan, studies of the exposure of young children in houses and childcare facilities were conducted following the aerial application of OP insecticides, including the volatile dichlorvos on rice using a remotely controlled helicopter. Inhalation exposure indoors at childcare facilities was comparable with, or more than, that at home and correlated inversely with the distance from the treated farm (Kawahara *et al.*, 2005).

In some areas of the world, and especially in tropical countries, residential areas are treated with insecticides to control mosquitoes and other vectors of disease. This can be in the form of a residual spray, a space treatment, or by sleeping under a treated bed-net. Residual sprays on the walls of dwellings with DDT wettable powder at 5 g/m^2 ai was the standard technique with compression sprayers to break the transmission of malaria during the 1950s. The technique is still used in areas with major malaria problems due to resistance of the parasite to drugs, such as chloroquine. However, the WHO has been promoting the use of treated bed-nets as a means of protecting young children from malaria. The nets can be treated by soaking the netting in a container with a suspension of a pyrethroid insecticide, but the trend is to use nets in which the insecticide is impregnated in the fibre before the net is manufactured. The residual activity of these 'perma-nets' is said to be five years, even when the nets are washed frequently, whereas the surface deposits on the locally treated nets is removed by washing. Risk assessments have shown that this technique is extremely safe for the occupants of the houses.

Other techniques such as the use of heated dispensers, mosquito coils and small aerosol dispensers are used by individual householders.

In some residential areas, insecticide is applied at a very low dose by fogging. Various types of thermal and cold foggers, either hand-carried or vehicle-mounted, may be deployed by health authorities. Crucially, the fog is applied only when the insects are actively flying. This timing will depend on the target vector, but it is usually in the evening or early morning. In the USA, although malaria is not a problem, mosquito control has been a major factor in areas such as Florida, where extensive wet areas provide ideal breeding sites for mosquitoes. Apart from a risk of exposure to encephalitis, the need for mosquito control has been emphasised in recent years by the spread across the USA of West Nile virus. Although known elsewhere, this virus was first detected in the USA in New York, following the death of many crows, and has spread to humans from birds by mosquito vectors. Despite the need to stop the disease spread, extensive use of space treatments with insecticide has caused concern.

In one study conducted in a park (Knepper *et al.*, 2003), a 20% permethrin plus 20% PBO formulation diluted 1:2 with water was applied at 0.0021 kg/ha ai as a cold fog. Filter papers placed on different surfaces were subsequently analysed to show that, after 12 hours post-treatment, there was a deposit of 0.66 ng/cm^2. The WHO ADI of permethrin is 0.05 mg/kg/day for the lifetime of an individual. If a child is playing in the park with a ball 28.2 cm diameter and half of the area picks up the permethrin residue from the surfaces on which it bounces, (i.e. a surface area of ca. 2500 cm^2) then the ball could pick up 827 ng. Assuming that all of this is transferred to the surface of a child's hand and 10% is absorbed through the skin, then the total amount of permethrin entering the child's body is calculated to be 82.7 ng. If the child weighed 25 kg, the exposure equals 3.3 ng/kg, which is over 15,000 times less than the ADI.

Thus, the very small dose used in these space treatments is not expected to cause any harm to children, and less so to adults.

In the developing countries, pesticides may be stored in houses, including the bedrooms, as this is considered one of the safest places to avoid theft (Fig. 5.12). The pesticides are sometimes purchased and stored in unlabelled containers (Ngowi *et al.*, 2001a; Matthews *et al.*, 2003). Unfortunately, medical services in rural areas do not have the required training in toxicity of pesticides and treatment in cases of poisoning (Ngowi *et al.*, 2001b).

Analysis for persistent insecticides in blood samples taken from 155 volunteers living in 13 different areas of the UK showed DDT still to be present, despite its use having been discontinued for many years. Blood samples also revealed the presence of other compounds, including PCBs (Table 5.1) (Anon, 2003).

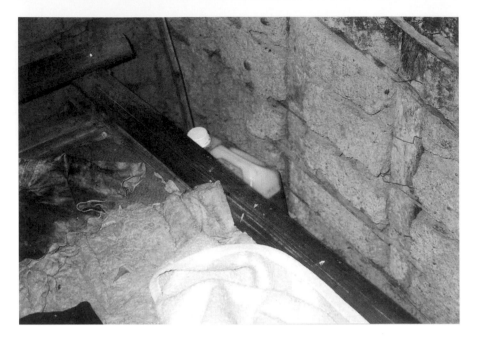

Fig. 5.12   Pesticide container in the bedroom of a house of an African villager.

Table 5.1   Chemical content of blood samples (ng/g lipid) in the United Kingdom, 2003

Chemical	Minimum	Maximum	Median
Total chemical	46	2024	360
Total DDT and metabolites	1.3	1715	107
Total organochlorine	7.1	1754	140
Total PCB*	14	665	169
Chemicals detected (n = 78)	9	49	27

*Brominated flame retardants are among the PCBs to which we are exposed.
Note: 1 ng = 0.000,000,001 g. While this quantity is extremely minute, it is at this nano level that reactions occur at the cellular level. DDT is stored in fatty tissues and has not been shown to affect man adversely following exposure to large quantities.

Worker exposure

Many people come into contact with surfaces treated with pesticides as part of their normal working day. These include those harvesting many crops and flowers, especially on protected cropping, where deposits may remain on foliage longer than when crops are exposed to rain. In particular, care is needed to avoid entry into and the touching of treated crops immediately after a spray application. Hands and other parts of the body that touch the treated surfaces may be wetted by spray deposits; alternatively, when the deposit has dried they may pick up dry, dislodgeable residues (Van Hemmen and Brouwer, 1997). The amount of dislodgeable residues is normally related to the dosage applied, but will be affected by the formulation used and the affinity of particles to the foliar surfaces. Their distribution will also be a function of the application technique. Exposure to these deposits is predominantly dermal and can also be intermittent; thus, from a toxicological point of view, Hakkert (2001) suggested setting more than one Acceptable Operator Exposure Level (AEOL) covering different periods of exposure.

Restricted entry intervals (REI) were first introduced in California to reduce the exposure of workers to pesticide residues on treated foliage. These were adopted elsewhere in the USA in accordance with Worker Protection Standards (Whitmyre *et al.*, 2005). Generally, these require a 48-, 24- or 12-hour restricted entry period, depending on the toxicity of the product applied. However, as the exposure to a low-toxicity product may be greater than to a high-toxicity pesticide, the trend is towards a risk assessment to determine the REI. This involves calculating a transfer coefficient (TC) that links the dislodgeable residue with the duration and type of exposure (e.g. touching leaves, fruit, flowers).

Assessments of the exposure of workers harvesting or otherwise touching treated plants is often by means of hand washing or skin wipes, using both chemical and mechanical action to transfer surface deposits to the sampling surface (Brouwer *et al.*, 2000c).

The methods are relatively inexpensive, but wipe sampling does not remove as much compared to hand-wash samples. Sampling is also influenced by the period between exposure and sampling, as the sample represents only what is still accessible to the sampling technique when this is done.

In a study in greenhouses in which chrysanthemums were being grown, dermal and inhalation exposure was measured during high-volume spray application of the OP insecticide methomyl. Subsequent studies using the fungicide chlorothalonil continued sampling for re-entry and harvesters (Brouwer *et al.*, 1994). The data provided a useful comparison of the exposure on hands during mixing the pesticide, spraying and either manually or automatic harvesting, which occurred on average 27 days after treatment (Table 5.2) to use in risk management. Inhalation exposure was generally less than 0.01 mg/h. Wearing gloves was shown to significantly lower actual exposure (Table 5.3) (Brouwer *et al.*, 2000a).

Other studies in Holland (Brouwer *et al.*, 1992) have examined cold fogging (called low-volume misting) in greenhouses. With the volume median diameter of droplets less than 50 µm, the threshold limit value of a volatile insecticide was still substantially exceeded 6 hours after application, but venting the greenhouse for 1 hour then permitted safe entry. Other glasshouse studies in California showed that a fog slowly settled during the night and re-admission was possible after venting (Giles *et al.*, 1995). The cold fogging

Table 5.2   Mean potential dermal exposure of the hands (from Brouwer *et al.*, 1994)

Exposure source	Exposure (mg/h)
Mixing and loading sprayer	13.0
During high-volume application	0.8
Harvesting	
Manual	3.6
Automatic	1.1

resulted in a more homogeneous distribution within the crop compared to high-volume spraying (Brouwer *et al.*, 2000b).

When comparing the impact of chemical pest management with an integrated pest management programme in two experimental greenhouses, Anton *et al.* (2004) considered that the selection of chemicals could be more important than choice of control programme in relation to life cycle assessment of pesticides, including human exposure routes.

If the average air concentration of an insecticide downwind of a crop being sprayed is 30 $\mu g/m^3$, over a 5-hour period, then reducing to 5 $\mu g/m^3$, the time-weighted average (TWA) is 10.2 $\mu g/m^3$. Thus, assuming a breathing rate of 15 m^3 per day, 100% absorption and a body weight of 60 kg, the exposure is 0.15 mg per person, or 0.002,55 mg/kg body weight per day. This value is then compared with the AOEL and ADI of the pesticide being considered. For a smaller person weighing only 25 kg, the exposure would be correspondingly higher at 0.006 mg/kg body weight per day, at the same breathing rate.

In risk assessment for those who may have to enter crops, and more generally in relation to the environment, registration authorities would like to have some indication of the amount of pesticide intercepted by a crop and the period over which deposits are retained. An attempt has been made to produce standardised values for foliar interception (Linders *et al.*, 2000), but the results will vary significantly between methods of application, the crop and subsequent weather conditions.

Table 5.3   Actual exposure of hands (in μg) to the insecticide propoxur.* Data expressed as median value and range (from Brouwer *et al.*, 2000a)

Operation	Gloves	No gloves
Mixing/loading	8 (7–148)	231 (8–5785)
Application	8 (4–47)	122 (9–416)
Total spraying	16 (11–56)	348 (31–2390)
Harvesters	8 (5–299)	164 (7–1523)

*Applied at 36.8 ± 14.3 g ai/1000 m^2 at an average volume rate of 113.5 ± 44.5 l/1000 m^2 over an average period of 36 min.

This chapter has provided information on the movement of spray from equipment, and how bystanders – and those living or working in areas where pesticides are used – may be exposed to the chemicals. The careful choice of pesticides, an avoidance of highly volatile chemicals, and changes in spray techniques, including the use of coarser sprays, shields and directed air-assisted sprayers – together termed drift reduction technology (DRT) – have reduced exposure to those who are not directly involved in the application processes. In some countries, buffer zones (see Chapter 6) are already required to protect sensitive areas, such as housing, schools and hospitals. With the reform of the Common Agricultural Policy, those farmers seeking the Single Farm Payment must 'set-aside' part of their arable land. The minimum width of land accepted as set-aside has been reduced from 10 to 5 m, so there should not be any impediment to these areas being buffer strips, provided that they are managed without spraying pesticides. Spot herbicide treatments to control certain weeds may still be required, however, in the buffer strip.

References

Anon (2003) *National Biomonitoring Survey.* WWF.

Anon (2004) *Pesticides Incidents Report 1 April 2003–31 March 2004.* HSE, Bootle.

Anton, A., Castells, F., Montero, J.I. and Huijbregts, M. (2004) Comparison of toxicological impacts of integrated and chemical pest management in Mediterranean greenhouses. *Chemosphere* **54**, 1225–1235.

Bernard, C.E., Nuygen, H., Truong, D. and Krieger, R.I. (2001) Environmental residues and biomonitoring estimates of human insecticide exposure from treated residential turf. *Archives of Environmental Contamination and Toxicology* **41**, 237–240.

Botella, B., Crespo, J., Rivas, A., Cerrillo, I., Olea-Serrano, M.F. and Olea, N. (2004) Exposure of women to organochlorine pesticides in Southern Spain. *Environmental Research* **96**, 34–40.

Bradman, M.A., Harnly, M.E., Draper, W., Seidel, S., Teran, S., Wakeham, D. and Neutra, R. (1997) Pesticide exposures to children from California's Central Valley: Results of a pilot study. *Journal of Exposure Analysis and Environmental Epidemiology* **7**, 217–234.

Briand, O., Bertrand, F., Seux, R. and Millet, M. (2002) Comparison of different sampling techniques for the evaluation of pesticide spray drift in apple orchards. *The Science of the Total Environment* **288**, 199–213.

Brouwer, D.H., de Vreede, J.A.F., Ravensberg, J.C., Engel, R. and van Hemmen, J.J. (1992) Dissipation of aerosols from greenhouse air after application of pesticides using a low volume technique. Implications for safe re-entry. *Chemosphere* **24**, 1157–1169.

Brouwer, D.H., de Vreede, J.A.F., de Haan, M., van der Vijver, L., Veerman, M., Stevenson, H. and van Hemmen, J.J. (1994) Exposure to pesticides during and after application in the cultivation of chrysanthemums in greenhouses. Health risk and risk management. *Med. Fac. Landbouww. University of Gent,* **59**, 3b.

Brouwer, D.H., Kroese, R. and van Hemmen, J.J. (1999) Transfer of contaminants from surface to hands: Experimental assessment of linearity of the exposure process, adherence to the skin and area exposed during fixed pressure and repeated contact with surfaces contaminated with powder. *Applied Occupational and Environmental Hygiene* **14**, 231–239.

Brouwer, D.H., Boeniger, M.F. and Van Hemmen, J. (2000a) Hand wash and manual skin wipes. *Annals of Occupational Health* **44**, 501–510.

Brouwer, D.H., de Haan, M. and van Hemmen, J.J. (2000b) Modelling re-entry exposure estimates. Application techniques and rates. In: Honeycutt, R.C., Day, E.W, Jr. (eds.), *Worker Exposure to Agrochemicals*. ACS Symposium Series. CRC Lewis Publishers, Baton Rouge, FL, USA, pp. 119–138.

Brouwer, D.H., de Vreede, S.A.F., Meuling, W.J.A. and van Hemmen, J.J. (2000c) Determination of the efficiency for pesticide exposure reduction with protective clothing: Field study using biological monitoring. In: Honeycutt, R.C., Day, E.W, Jr. (eds.), *Worker Exposure to Agrochemicals*. ACS Symposium Series. CRC Lewis Publishers, Baton Rouge, FL, USA, pp. 63 –84.

Cross, J.V., Walklare, P.J., Murray, R.A. and Richardson, G.M. (2001) Spray deposits and losses in different sized apple trees from an axial fan orchard sprayer: 1. Effects of spray liquid flow rate. *Crop Protection* **20**, 13– 30.

DEFRA (2003) Report on bystander exposure trials [unpublished].

Dobson, C.M., Minski, M.J. and Matthews, G.A. (1983) Neutron activation analysis using dysprosium as a tracer to measure spray drift. *Crop Protection* **2**, 345–352.

Driver, J.H. and Whitmyre, G.K. (1996) Assessment of residential exposures to pesticides and other chemicals. *Pesticide Outlook* **7**, 6–10.

Driver, J., Ross, J.H., Pandian, M., Evans, J. and Lunchick, C. (2005) Residential (non-dietary) post-application exposure assessment. In: Franklin, C.A. and Worgan, J.P. (eds.), *Occupational and Residential Exposure Assessment for Pesticides*. Wiley, Chichester, pp. 129–170.

Elliott, J.G. and Wilson, B.J. (1983) *The Influence of Weather on the Efficiency and Safety of Pesticide Application: The drift of herbicides*. BCPC Occasional Publication 3.

Epple, J., Maguhn, J., Spitzauer, P. and Kettrup, A. (2002) Input of pesticides by atmospheric deposition. *Geoderma* **105**, 327–349.

Garry, V. F. (2004) Pesticides and children. *Toxicology and Applied Pharmacology* **198**, 152–163.

Gilbert, A.J. and Bell, G.J. (1988) Evaluation of the drift hazards arising from pesticide spray application. *Aspects of Applied Biology* **17**, 363–376.

Giles, D.K., Welsh, A., Steinke, W.E. and Saiz, S.G. (1995) Pesticide inhalation exposure, air concentration and droplet size spectra from greenhouse fogging. *Transactions of the ASAE* **38**, 1321–1326.

Grey, C.N.B., Nieuwenhuijsen, M.J., Golding, J. and the ALSPAC Team (2004). The use and disposal of household pesticides. *Environmental Research* **97**, 109–115.

Grover, R., Maybank, J. and Yoshida, K. (1972) Droplet and vapor drift from butyl ester and dimethylamine salt of 2,4-D. *Weed Science* **20**, 320–324.

Hakkert, B.C. (2001) Refinement of risk assessment of dermally and intermittently exposed pesticide workers: A critique. *Annals of Occupational Health* **45**, S23–S28.

Harrad, S. and Mao, H. (2004) Atmospheric PCBs and organochlorine pesticides in Birmingham, UK: Concentrations, sources, temporal and seasonal trends. *Atmospheric Environment* **38**, 1437–1445.

Hatfield, J.L., Wesley, C.K., Prueger, J.H. and Pfeiffer, R.L. (1996) Herbicide and nitrate distribution in Central Iowa rainfall. *Journal of Environmental Quality* **25**, 259–264.

Himel, C.M. (1974) Analytical methodology in ULV. *British Crop Protection Monograph* **11**, 112–119.

Johnstone, D.R. and Matthews, G.A. (1965) Evaluation of swath pattern and droplet size provided by a boom and nozzle installation fitted to a Hiller UH-12 helicopter. *Agricultural Aviation* **7**(2), 46–50.

Kawahara, J., Horikoshi, R., Yamaguchi, T., Kumagai, K. and Yaragisawa, Y. (2005) Air pollution and young children's inhalation exposure to organophosphorus pesticide in an agricultural community in Japan. *Environmental International* **31**, 1123–1132.

Knepper, R.G., Walker, E.D. and Kamrin, M.A. (2003) ULV studies of permethrin in Saginaw, Michigan. *Wing Beats*, **14**, 22–23, 32–33.

Krieger, R.I., Dinoff, T.M. and Ross, J.H. (2001) Pesticide exposure assessment: Jazzercize™ activities to determine extreme case indoor exposure potential and in-use biomonitoring. In: Honeycutt, R.C. and Day, E.W. (eds.), *Worker Exposure to Agrochemicals*. CRC Lewis Publishers, Boca Raton, FL, USA, pp. 97–106.

Lee, S., McLaughlin, R., Harnly, M., Gunier, R. and Kreutzer, R. (2002) Community exposures to airborne agricultural pesticides in California: Ranking of inhalation risks. *Environmental Health Perspectives* **110**, 1175–1184.

Linders, J., Mensink, H., Stephenson, G., Wauchope, D. and Racke, K. (2000) Foliar interception and retention values after pesticide application. A proposal for standardized values for environmental risk assessment. *Pure and Applied Chemistry* **72**, 2199–2218.

Lloyd, G.A., Bell, G.J., Samuels, S.W., Cross, J.V. and Berrie, A.M. (1987) *Orchard Sprayers: Comparative operator exposure and spray drift study*. MAFF Report.

Lu, C. and Fenske, R.A. (1999) Dermal transfer of chlorpyrifos residues from residential surfaces: Comparison of hand press, hand drag, wipe and polyurethane foam roller measurements after broadcast and aerosol pesticide applications. *Environmental Health Perspectives* **107**, 463–467.

Lu, C., Fenske, R.A., Simcox, N.J. and Kalman, D. (2000) Pesticide exposure of children in an agricultural community: Evidence of household proximity to farmland and take home exposure pathways. *Environmental Research Section* **A84**, 290–302

Lu, C., Kedan, G., Fisker-Andersen, J., Kissel, J.C. and Fenske, R.A. (2004) Multipathway organophosphorus pesticide exposures of pre-school children living in agricultural and non-agricultural communities. *Environmental Research* **96**, 283–289.

Mason, M.A, Sheldon, I.S. and Stout, D.M., II (2000) The distribution of chlorpyrifos in air, carpeting and dust and its reemission from carpeting following the use of total release aerosols in an indoor air quality test house. *Proceedings of the Symposium on Engineering Solutions to Indoor Air Quality Problems*. Raleigh, NC, 17–19 July, pp. 92–102.

Matthews, G.A. and Johnstone, D.R. (1968) Aircraft and tractor spray deposits on irrigated cotton. *Cotton Growers Review* **45**, 207–218.

Matthews, G.A., Wiles, T. and Baleguel, P. (2003) A survey of pesticide application in Cameroon. *Crop Protection* **22**, 707–714.

Miller, P.C.H, (1993) Spray Drift and its Measurement In Matthews and Hislop E.C. *Application Technology for Crop Protection*. CABI Wallingford 101–122.

Muir, K., Rattanamongkolgl, S., Smallman-Raynor, M., Thomas, M., Downer, S. and Jenkinson, C. (2004) Breast cancer incidence and its possible spatial association with pesticide application in two counties of England. *Public Health* **118**, 513–520.

Neumann, M., Schulz, R., Schafer, K., Muller, W., Mannheller, W. and Liess, M. (2002) The significance of entry routes as point and non-point sources of pesticides in small streams. *Water Research* **36**, 835–842.

Ngowi, A.V.F., Maeda, D.N., Wesseling, C., Partenen, T.J., Sanga, M.P. and Mbise, G. (2001a) Pesticide-handling practices in agriculture in Tanzania: Observational data from 27 coffee and cotton farms. *International Journal of Occupational and Environmental Health* **7**, 326–332.

Ngowi, A.V.F., Maeda, D.N. and Partenen, T.J. (2001b) Assessment of the ability of health care providers to treat and prevent adverse health effects of pesticides in agricultural areas of Tanzania. *International Journal of Occupational and Environmental Health* **7**, 349–356.

Piggott, S.J. and Matthews, G.A. (1999) Air induction nozzles: A solution to spray drift? *International Pest Control* **41**, 24–28.

Ramaprasad, J., Tsai, M.-Y., Elgetthun, K., Hebert, V.R., Felsot, A., Yost, M.G. and Fenske, R.A. (2004) The Washington aerial spray drift study: Assessment of off-target organophosphorus insecticide atmospheric movement by plant surface volatilization. *Atmospheric Environment* **38**, 5703–5713.

Reynolds, P., Hurley, S.E., Goldberg, D.E., Yerabati, S., Gunier, R.B., Hertz, A., Anton-Culver, H., Berstein, L., Deapen, D., Horn-Ross, P.L., Peel, D., Pinder, R., Ross, R.K., West, D., Wright, W.E. and Ziogas, A. (2004) Residential proximity to agricultural pesticide use and incidence of breast cancer in the California Teachers Study cohort. *Environmental Research* **96**, 206–218.

Roff, M., Baldwin, P., Thompson, J. and Wheeler, J. (1998) Consumer exposure arising from the application of indoor pesticides. *Journal of Aerosol Science* **29**, S1291–S1292.

Scheyer, A., Graeff, C., Morville, S., Mirabel, P. and Millet, M. (2005) Analysis of some organochlorine pesticides in an urban atmosphere (Strasbourg, east of France). *Chemosphere* **58**, 1517–1524.

Schulz, R. (2001) Comparison of spray drift and run off-related input of azinphos-methyl and endosulfan from fruit orchards into the Lourens river, South Africa. *Chemosphere* **45**, 543–551.

Siebers, J., Binner, R. and Wittich, K.-P. (2003) Investigation on downwind short-range transport of pesticides after application in agricultural crops. *Chemosphere* **51**, 397–407.

Stoughton, T.E., Miller, D.R., Yang, X. and Ducharme, K.M. (1997) A comparison of spray drift predictions to lidar data. *Agricultural and Forest Meteorology* **88**, 15–26.

Stout, D.M., II and Mason, M.A. (2003) The distribution of chlorpyrifos following a crack and crevice type application in the US EPA Indoor Air Quality Research House. *Atmospheric Environment* **37**, 5539–5549.

Teil, M.-J., Blanchard, M. and Chevreuil, M. (2004) Atmospheric deposition of orga-nochlorines (PCBs and pesticides) in northern France. *Chemosphere* **55**, 501–504.

Turnbull, A B. (1995) *An assessment of the fate and behaviour of selected pesticides in rural England.* PhD thesis, University of Birmingham.

Unsworth, J.B., Wauchope, R.D., Klein, A.W., Dorn, E., Zeeh, B., Yeh, S.M., Akerblom, M., Racke, K.D. and Rubin, B. (1999) Significance of the long range transport of pesticides in the atmosphere. *Pure and Applied Chemistry* **71**, 1359–1383.

Van Hemmen, J.J. and Brouwer, D.H. (1997) Exposure assessment for pesticides: Operators and harvesters risk evaluation and risk management. *Med. Fac. Landbouww. University of Gent* **62/2**, 113–130.

Whitmyre, G.K., Ross, J.H., Ginevan, M.E. and Eberhart, D. (2005) Development of risk-based restricted entry intervals. In: Franklin, C.A. and Worgan, J.P. (eds.), *Occupational and Residential Exposure Assessment for Pesticides.* Wiley, Chichester, pp. 45–69.

6 Environmental aspects of spray drift

In addition to the concerns about pesticides affecting the human population directly, registration authorities are also concerned with more general effects in the environment on other non-target organisms, which can also have indirect effects on people.

Protecting water

A major consideration in protecting the environment from exposure to pesticides has been to minimise spray droplets drifting and subsequently sedimenting on water surfaces. Many of the studies on spray drift (as referred to in Chapter 5) have concentrated on the amount of pesticide collected on flat sampling surfaces within a relatively short distance downwind, rather than measurements of airborne drift. Studies in Germany (Ganzelmeier *et al.*, 1995; Ganzelmeier and Rautmann, 2000) and others (e.g. Hewitt, 2000) have provided data to support legislation requiring no-spray or 'buffer' zones, the width of which depends on the type of pesticide and risk assessments in relation to fish and other aquatic organisms (Fig. 6.1). It also takes account of the need to minimise exposure so that water extracted for drinking meets the EU standards, namely 0.1 µg/l for a single pesticide and 0.5 µg/l for all pesticides. There is also a standard of 0.03 µg/l for certain pesticides.

Studies by de Snoo and de Wit (1998) confirmed that the amount of pesticide deposited in ditches (Fig. 6.2) was affected by the choice of nozzle and wind speed. They concluded that with a 6-m buffer zone, no deposition was recorded in a ditch when the wind speed was 4.5 m/s, and therefore having unsprayed crop edges offered a good way of protecting aquatic ecosystems.

In the UK, farmers were not keen to lose 6 m around the edges of their fields. In view of developments in spray technology, it was decided that a narrower buffer zone would be acceptable if the method of application and/or dose of pesticide applied was adjusted. This led to the Local Environmental Risk Assessment for Pesticides (LERAP) being developed (Gilbert, 2000) (Table 6.1). Farms have as many as 75% of their fields alongside watercourses, so the adoption of LERAP is important. In arable crops, many

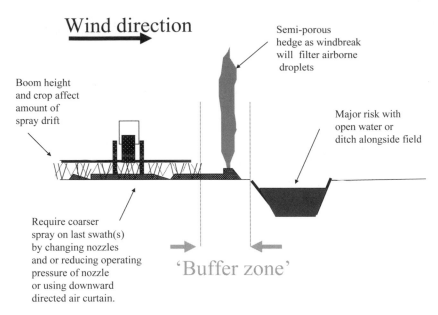

Wind direction

Semi-porous
hedge as windbreak
will filter airborne
droplets

Boom height
and crop affect
amount of
spray drift

Major risk with
open water or
ditch alongside field

Require coarser
spray on last swath(s)
by changing nozzles
and or reducing operating
pressure of nozzle
or using downward
directed air curtain.

'Buffer zone'

Fig. 6.1 Diagram showing the position of a buffer zone to protect a watercourse.

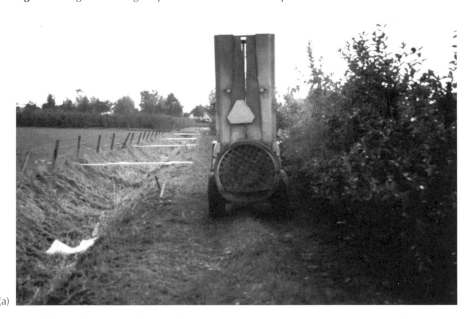

(a)

Fig. 6.2 (a) Measuring drift into a ditch. (*Continued.*)

farmers have adopted the use of LERAP 3* nozzles, usually air-induction
nozzles, to reduce the potential drift and allow the width of buffer zones
to be reduced. In practice, farmers tend to use the 3* nozzle over the whole
field, whereas they could use a more suitable nozzle over much of the crop

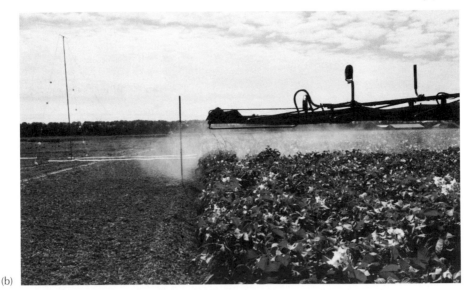

(b)

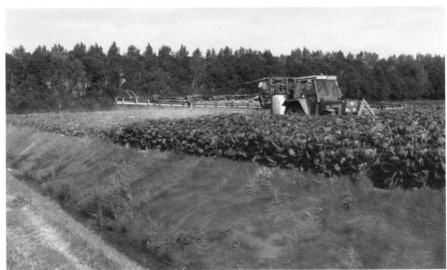

(c)

Fig. 6.2 (*Continued.*) (b,c) Measuring drift in Holland (illustrations courtesy of Jan van der Zande).

Table 6.1 LERAP calculations to determine minimum width of buffer zone (m) from top of the bank for arable crops, with or without 3* nozzle rating

Width of watercourse	Full dose as on label		¾ dose	
	No star	***	No star	***
<3 m	5	1	4	1
3–6 m	3	1	2	1
>6 m	2	1	1	1
Dry ditch	1	1	1	1

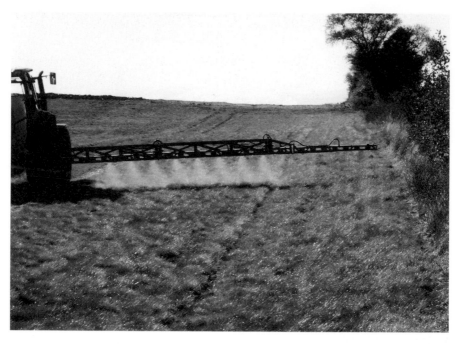

Fig. 6.3   Avoiding spraying from nozzles at the edge of the boom in order to reduce drift of spray into the hedge (photograph Hardi International).

and change to the coarser spray for the last downwind swaths across the field nearest to a watercourse or ditch. Drift can be reduced by shutting off nozzles when close to the field boundary (Fig. 6.3), ensuring that the boom is not set too high (Fig. 6.4) and checking the wind speed to ensure it is within the recommended limits (Fig. 6.5), or changing the nozzle (Fig. 6.6). There is a trend to increase tractor speeds as well as increase boom width, but more air turbulence is created behind the tractor at the faster speeds (Fig. 6.7).

Where lower doses are used they must be used over the whole treated area. In the UK, air is usually sufficiently moist [$\Delta T < 7^{\circ}C$), but in arid areas low humidity can increase evaporation from droplets. As droplets shrink in volume they are more likely to remain airborne and drift further (Parkin *et al.*, 2003). Actual drift will also be affected by the formulation and concentration at which it is applied (Butler Ellis and Bradley, 2002). Herbst (2003), using vertical collectors in a wind tunnel to calculate a drift potential index (DIX), reported that using a particular air-induction nozzle, the drift potential was 50% compared with a flat-fan nozzle (F110/1.2/3.0); however, when the herbicide glyphosate was used, the drift potential was only reduced by just over 25%. This may have been due to the formulation affecting the surface tension of the spray liquid and thus the break up of the liquid sheet. Adoption of buffer zones would be greater if there was a financial incentive, for example by allowing narrow strips to be eligible as set-aside areas.

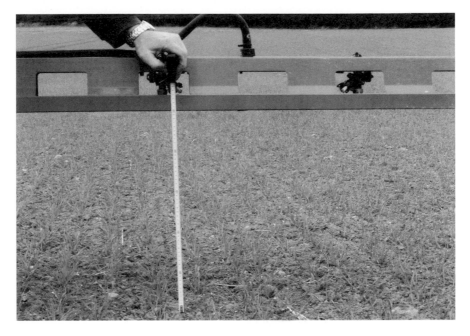

Fig. 6.4 Checking the boom height to avoid a too-high boom causing more downwind drift (photograph Hardi International).

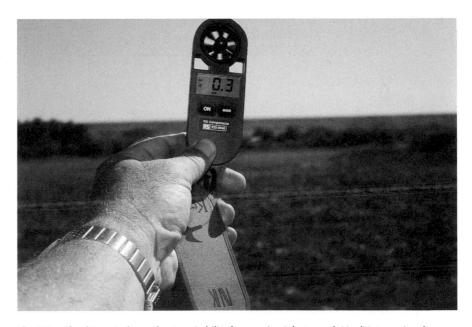

Fig. 6.5 Checking wind speed as to suitability for spraying (photograph Hardi International).

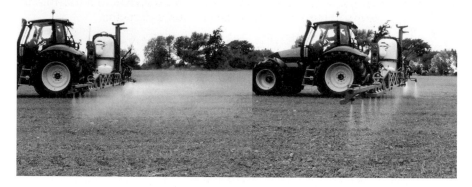

Fig. 6.6   Changing the nozzle or reducing pressure to reduce drift (photograph Hardi International).

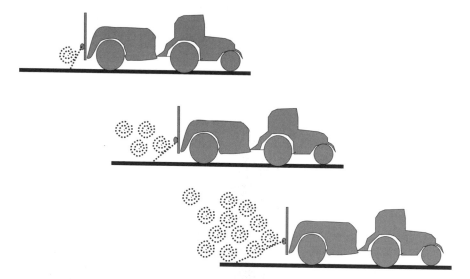

Fig. 6.7   Higher tractor speeds create more turbulence, causing (potentially) more drift behind the tractor.

In Germany, maps have been made of rivers and their tributaries so that, by using a GIS-based decision support system with a graphical user interface, a farmer can determine where he or she can treat their fields without infringing the regulations to protect water (Ropke *et al.*, 2004; Ganzelmeier, 2005) (Fig. 6.8).

A similar LERAP system operates for orchards, but as the risk of drift is greater, the minimum buffer zone is 5 m, even with tunnel sprayers. Those treating orchards are in a more difficult situation as spray is directed upwards into and over tree canopies. Complex interactions between the air passing

Minimum distance of an agricultural field to the nearest water body

Converting surface water and field geometry from ATKIS in a GIS-raster format with a pixel (cell) resolution of 5 meter

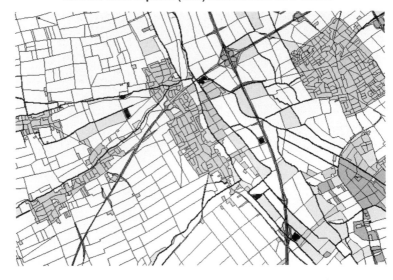

(a)

Minimum distance of an agricultural field to the nearest water body

Calculating for each cell the distance (Euclidean distance) to the nearest water body

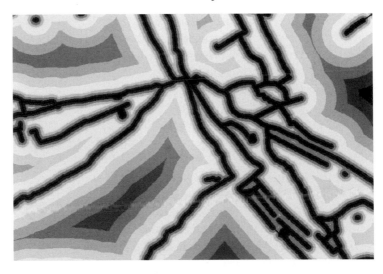

(b)

Fig. 6.8　Using GPS and GIS in Germany to protect rivers (Ganzelmeier Germany). Different sources of pesticide affecting water sources. (a) Map of the area; (b) calculating distances from the water courses. (*Continued.*)

through and over the orchard with the airflow from the sprayer occur, so that droplet movement is much more difficult to predict compared with field crops. In some cases droplets travel in the opposite direction to the cross-

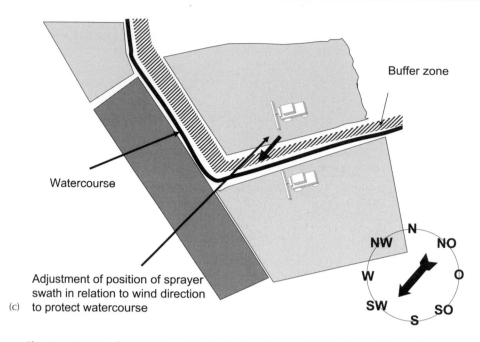

Buffer zone

Watercourse

Adjustment of position of sprayer
swath in relation to wind direction
(c)   to protect watercourse

N
NW   NO
W   O
SW   SO
S

Fig. 6.8   *(Continued.)* (c) Position of the tractor in relation to wind direction and strength.

flow (Farooq *et al.*, 2001). Typically, an undirected axial fan has been used on orchard sprayers, while for some pesticides very wide buffer zones were needed. In bioassay tests, insect mortality of 10% was recorded at about 50 m downwind of orchard spraying (Davis *et al.*, 1994a). Many orchards are protected by wind-breaks of alder and other plants, and these act as filters to reduce downwind drift. Such a filter needs to be sufficiently porous to allow air flow yet have sufficient foliage to collect the spray droplets. Thus, the efficiency in terms of filtering improves in late spring and early summer as the amount of foliage increases. In practice, a farmer needs to be careful which pesticides are used to avoid killing beneficial insects that survive in the wind-breaks. If a wind-break is too solid then air-flows tend to go over the top of the wind-break or hedge. In one study there was a sudden decrease in deposition in the shelter of the hedge, followed by a gradual increase over the next 15 m, a distance equivalent to nine-times the hedge height (Davis *et al.*, 1994b). Whilst a hedge and vegetation along streams will protect a watercourse downwind (Dabrowski *et al.*, 2005), smaller droplets carried by the airflow will be filtered on insects and vegetation over a longer distance.

Some sprays have been adapted with shields to minimise drift (e.g. Sidahmed *et al.*, 2004), while others have enclosed the trees in a mobile 'tunnel' while spraying. Growing smaller trees in trellises facilitates some of these newer sprayers. In some situations with flat land, the use of a 'tunnel' sprayer enables spray that penetrates through the crop canopy to be collected on the tunnel wall and to be re-circulated (Fig. 6.9). While drift can be reduced, uniformity of deposit on tree canopies is more difficult to

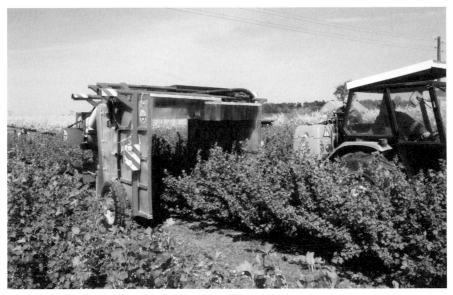

(a)

(b)

Fig. 6.9   Tunnel sprayer enclosing nozzles to reduce drift (a) in vines and (b) in apples (photograph from Greg Doruchowski, Poland).

achieve unless the nozzles are correctly adjusted relative to the tree profile (Planas *et al.*, 2002).

In the UK, a system using pictograms for pesticide dosage adjustment in relation to the crop environment (PACE) for apple orchard spraying with axial-fan equipment takes account of different tree sizes and canopy density (Fig. 6.10) (Cross *et al.*, 2004). Reductions in the pesticide dose can be taken into account as a factor when using a LERAP, and may allow a reduction in buffer zone widths.

In practice, spray drift is not the main source of contamination in water. In many cases the most serious cases of pesticide pollution are due to spillages, especially of the undiluted pesticide, run-off from surface deposits and the washing out of equipment, especially if this is done on hard surfaces (Figs. 6.11 and 6.12). One example of these problems is the use of herbicides in urban areas to keep gutters free of weeds along the edges of roads, although the washing out of sprayers on concrete farmyards has also led to chemicals being washed into drains. This is most obvious if heavy rain occurs soon after an application. Single rainfall events, which resulted in run-off, caused the most non-point source pollution in a catchment studied in Germany (Muller *et al.*, 2003). In monitoring a single drain outfall from a field with clay soil, 99% of the pesticide, sulfosulfuron, loading to the drain occurred in the first 12.5 mm of flow within 14 days of treatment, and represented 0.5% of the herbicide applied to the 7.7-ha site (Brown *et al.*, 2004a).

PACE dose adjustments for reduced tree area density

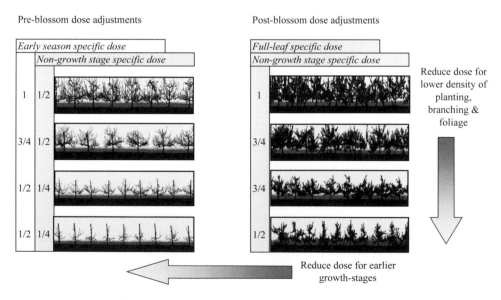

Fig. 6.10 Using PACE to decide on spray dosage (courtesy Peter Walklate, Silsoe Research Institute).

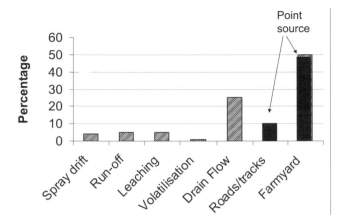

Fig. 6.11   Sources of pesticide pollution in water.

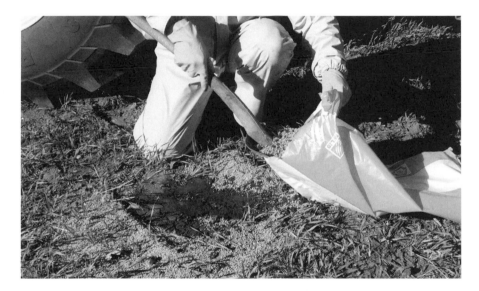

Fig. 6.12   Pesticide spilt on the ground is removed for safe disposal (photograph Hardi International).

Peak levels of pesticide in river water samples, caused by surface run-off following storms involving 6.8–18.4 mm rain per day, were from two to forty-one times higher than the levels recorded due to spray drift (0.04–0.07 μg/l), even when the river discharge rate was much greater (7–22.4 m³/s instead of 0.28 m³/s) (Schultz, 2001). In Germany, 24 g of pesticides were found in each farmyard run-off during the application period, presumably caused by cleaning of the spraying equipment (Neumann *et al.*, 2002). This has led to the need for an additional water tank on the sprayer so at least the inside of the tank is washed in the field and the washings are used to spray the last part of a field. A new International Standard for sprayer washing (ISO22368 parts 1–3) has also been published

Similar rapid loss of herbicides following application to the kerbside of roads during the first rainfall event was reported by Ramwell *et al.* (2002), and of an insecticide applied to turf (Armbrust and Peeler, 2002), but not from railway tracks treated with herbicide (Ramwell *et al.*, 2004). In fact, the impact of pesticides in urban areas can be higher than in neighbouring agricultural areas. Thus, the highest concentration of diuron in a French catchment area was 8.7 µg/l due to its application on hard surfaces (Blanchoud *et al.*, 2004); this level was far in excess of the EU drinking water standards. In Germany, non-agricultural use of pesticides contributed more than two-thirds of the pesticide load in tributaries and at least one-third in the River Ruhr (Skark *et al.*, 2004). Even quite low concentrations of pesticides, such as greater than 0.01-fold acute toxicity to *Daphnia* (49-h LC_{50}), affected the macro-invertebrate community structure in agricultural streams due to run-off (Berenzen *et al.*, 2005a). This emphasises the need for safety factors in assessing the registration of pesticides.

In California, where there is a tax on pesticides of 2.1% of wholesale value, one suggestion was that there should be an increase to 10% for three years to generate extra funds to support educational programmes for growers on how to reduce the volume of, or eliminate, pesticide run-off. Those growers who enrolled for training would get an incentive by receiving a rebate that would compensate for the increased tax (*IPM News*, May 2005).

When rain washes deposits from the crops, apart from reduced efficacy it also contributes to water pollution. Schultz (2001) reported rainfall-induced run-off from orchards following a storm that precipitated 28.8 mm of rain. Increased concentrations of several pesticides were detected, with some extremely high levels that exceeded national water quality standards. The effects persisted for about 3.5 months, thus illustrating that a short-term exposure has the potential of longer-term effects. A simple model to predict pesticide run-off in many streams on a landscape level has been proposed where limited data are available (Berenzen *et al.*, 2005b). A concern is that where farmers adopt air-induction nozzles to reduce spray drift, there could be more endo-drift on the soil surface to contribute to run-off. Run-off following rain is also reported to be increased where crops are covered by plastic covers or mulches (Arnold *et al.*, 2004).

Run-off rates of 8–22% of nine herbicides from rice paddies studied in Japan showed a correlation with the octanol-water partition coefficient log P_{ow} rather than the water solubility of the herbicides (Nakano *et al.*, 2004).

In developing countries, there are few relevant data available, but Tariq *et al.* (2003) detected several locally used pesticides in open wells in Pakistan, that were used as rural water supplies. In this particular case the maximum concentration levels established by the US EPA were not exceeded. However, in India, Sankararamakrishnan *et al.* (2004) reported high concentrations of organochlorine and organophosphate pesticides in surface and ground waters, with the concentration of malathion being much higher than the EC water quality standards. Ecological monitoring methods for the assessment of the impact of pesticides in the tropics have been published (Grant and Tingle, 2002), together with guides for practical field assessments.

Pollution of water due to pesticides also needs to be put into the context of other pollutants, some of natural origin. Sampling directly under areas of bracken, for example, shows that a carcinogenic water-soluble substance ptaquiloside can be detected at 7 µg/l at a depth of 90 cm. Fortunately, this compound is unstable under both acidic and alkaline conditions and will transform to pterosin B, which is harmless (Rasmussen *et al.*, 2003).

In the UK, water is sampled in many locations and at frequent intervals to meet the EU Directives on water quality, the data being kept at the Toxic and Persistent Substances (TAPS) Centre. The Environment Agency publishes a summary of the data, which shows where surface water and groundwater contain pesticide concentrations that exceed the 0.1 µg/l limit. Pesticides that exceed the limit are usually herbicides, from large-scale use on farms, but exceedances may also be related to urban use. Guidelines are also available for example for those farmers dipping sheep and who have to dispose safely quantities of pesticide-containing water from the dip (Anon, 2001). A number of computer models have been developed to assist with assessing the amount of pesticide in water. SWATCATCH is one model that can simulate maximum concentrations of pesticide at different times in surface waters (Brown *et al.*, 2002).

In the USA, water is similarly sampled under the National Water-Quality Assessment (NAWQA) Program of the US Geological Survey. Between 1993 and 1995, data were obtained from 2227 sites (wells and springs) sampled in twenty major hydrologic basins across the United States. Six herbicides were detected in shallow groundwater, but overall more than 98% of the detections during the NAWQA investigations were at concentrations of less than 1 µg/l, and this standard was exceeded at fewer than 0.1% of the sites. All of these exceedances involved atrazine. Of the sites sampled during the survey, two or more herbicides could be detected only at fewer than 20% of the sites.

One inevitable outcome of contamination of water is that of possible adverse effects on the populations of fish and other aquatic organisms, especially the crustacea and molluscs. The activity of the botanical insecticide rotenone was first noted when used traditionally to stun fish, which were then easy to net. Not surprisingly, major fish kills followed the use of highly toxic insecticides in lowland irrigated rice paddies. This is a particular problem where fish farms are located alongside irrigated land, as in many parts of Asia. Endosulfan is particularly toxic to fish, such as Nile tilapia (*Oreochromis niloticus*) (Cagauan, 1995) and can persist in paddy water and soil for up to 73 days after spraying, although microbial activity does cause degradation.

In contrast to agricultural use where whole fields were treated, studies on the impact of DDT used to control tsetse flies in Zimbabwe, where deposits were localised to tsetse resting sites, indicated no fish kills in the Kariba area. However, residues of DDT and metabolites were higher in fish sampled in sprayed areas with seasonal rivers flowing into the Zambezi, compared to unsprayed areas. These fish were considered to be a source of contamination for fish-eating birds, such as the fish eagle (Douthwaite and Tingle, 1994). Detailed ecotoxicological studies were also conducted in Botswana, where aerial sprays of a low dose of 6–12 g/ha endosulfan was applied as an aerosol of droplets smaller than about 70 µm against tsetse flies in the Okavambo swamp (Fox and Matthiessen, 1982). Careful application of sequential drift sprays resulted in concentrations of 0.2 to 4.2 µg/l in water at 6–9 h after spraying. The apparent mortality of fish varied from 0 to 60%, but high kills were sporadic and possibly caused by leaks from the equipment. Overall, only a few small fish were affected, with an average of 0–4% mortality per cycle depending on the species. Later, the use of deltamethrin was seen to be safer for fish, although it affected more arthropods in tree canopies. This was due to pyrethroid insecticides being adsorbed onto soil particles suspended in the water.

While on most occasions the aim is to prevent pesticides from reaching the water, some situations occur where the water must be treated with pesticides. These include the application of insecticides as larvicides to control the immature stages of important vectors of human diseases, notably anopheline mosquito vectors of malaria and other mosquitoes, as well as *Simulium* spp., the black fly vector of onchocerciasis that causes infected people to become blind. In most cases, preference is now given to *Bacillus thuringiensis israelensis* (Bti), although the organophosphate insecticide temephos, the pyrethroid permethrin and some insect growth regulators such as pyriproxyfen are used. In some cases herbicides used to control algae and waterweeds, such as water hyacinth, will also require direct application to water surfaces.

Recently, concern has been expressed that some pesticides and their metabolites may remain in the environment bound to soil, and are not extracted by the usual chemical processes. These residues may be so tightly bound that they are essentially not available, but some researchers have postulated that if the load of these chemicals were to build up, a time may come when they might be released. The risk of future problems is difficult to assess but, for single additions of individual pesticides, their binding to the soil seems to provide an environmental solution to the problem (Barraclough *et al.*, 2005). The situation is less clear where different compounds are involved with multiple residues.

Protecting vegetation

Reduction in drift is also crucial to protect plants downwind of treated areas. Much of the attention to drift was initiated when horticultural crops were damaged by a volatile herbicide that had been applied to control broad-leaved weeds in cereals (Elliott and Wilson, 1983). Koch *et al.* (2004a) have illustrated, by using paraquat herbicide, that the effect of the large droplets that sediment rapidly is clear-cut and limited, although there can be a short downwind displacement of the spray. However, the airborne droplets, when affected by surface friction and turbulence, cause trails of drift that influence their distribution and subsequent effects downwind. With paraquat, further downwind effects are shown by individual droplets scorching the leaves. This illustrates the difference between laboratory studies using low doses of pesticide in relatively high volumes to assess effects on non-target species, with the reality of a patchy distribution of a very low volume of liquid in small droplets, containing a higher concentration of pesticide (Koch *et al.*, 2004b). In consequence, an alternative to the laboratory investigation was suggested by Koch and Weisser (2004). The ability of plants outside crops to survive complete kill and still produce seeds is crucial, not only from the point of view of plant biodiversity, but also as a source of seeds for birds and other non-target organisms.

Exposure to non-target terrestrial organisms and the plants on which they can forage has been estimated using the standard drift data developed by Ganzelmeier *et al.* (1995), but as this is mainly concerned with deposition on the ground at different distances downwind, it can significantly under-estimate the true exposure (Lane and Butler-Ellis, 2003). Most drift studies were always over open ground, but edges of fields have hedges and other vegetation which affects the air flow (Figs. 6.13 and 6.14). Individual plants in a hedge not only provide a vertical barrier, but will also filter out some of the droplets that are airborne and still large enough to impact on leaves and stems, rather than continue to be carried in the air flow. Thus, non-target organisms within the hedge can be affected by the drift collected there.

When studying the effect of drift in relation to a hedge and effect of gaps in a hedge, Davis *et al.* (1993) used various sampling surfaces to detect a fluorescent tracer, and also assessed the impact of the herbicide MCPA on seedlings of ragged-robin (*Lychnis flos-cuculi*). The results were confirmed by similar bioassays with an insect, and showed that the area immediately behind the hedge was protected from the spray, whereas 13 m behind the hedge there was little or no difference from results obtained where there was a gap in the hedge.

As a follow-up of studies in relation to protecting water in ditches, de Snoo and van der Poll (1999) showed that alongside the edges of wheat fields that were not sprayed to leave a buffer zone, the diversity and cover of dicotyledons increased, enhancing the floristic value of the vegetation.

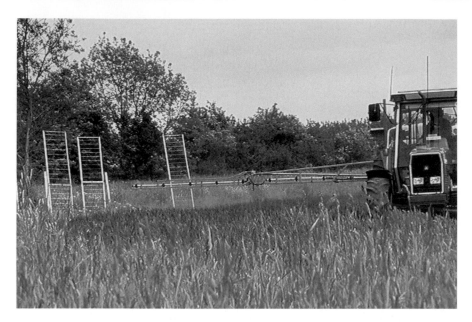

Fig. 6.13   Measuring drift adjacent to a hedgerow (courtesy Paul Miller, Silsoe Research Institute).

Similar changes were not significant alongside potato or sugar-beet, probably because of differences in herbicide use. De Snoo (1999) pointed out that, from a farming perspective, it is important to have flexibility in the width of unsprayed crop edges. In Canada, a vegetated 10-m field margin provided protection from herbicide drift into a wetland area under wind conditions normally acceptable for spraying, but in high winds this needs to be extended to 20 m, unless there is also a windbreak with a porosity of 25% (Brown *et al.*, 2004b). Some porosity is essential, otherwise the wind will take any droplets up and over the barrier. Using a probabilistic model to assess risk to organisms in an aquatic environment with chlorpyrifos as an example being sprayed on top fruit, 5% of TER values will be less than 1, even with a buffer zone of 80 m. Thus, the EC_{50} for randomly selected arthropod species will be exceeded after 5% of spray events with this wide a buffer zone (Crane *et al.*, 2003).

Using LIDAR equipment, Miller and Stoughton (2000) showed that, when an aerial spray was applied to the edge of a hardwood forest, small droplets were dispersed in the atmospheric boundary layer. The implication was that even with well-conducted spray operations a small amount of pesticide will be widely dispersed. However, where bracken has to be controlled by applying a herbicide, asulam, aerially in inaccessible areas, such as hillsides, on which a farmer wishes to graze sheep, drift from 'Raindrop' drift reducing hollow cone nozzles on a helicopter was mainly limited to 35 m downwind. Drift beyond 35 m of the treated area was similar to the drift from ground

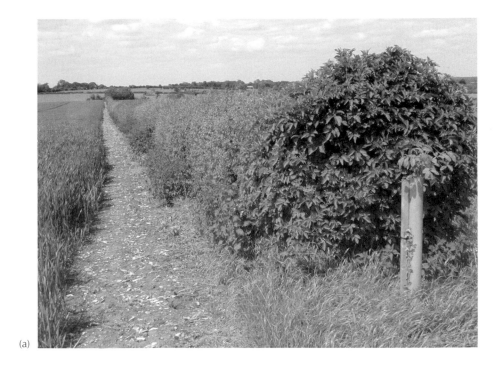

(a)

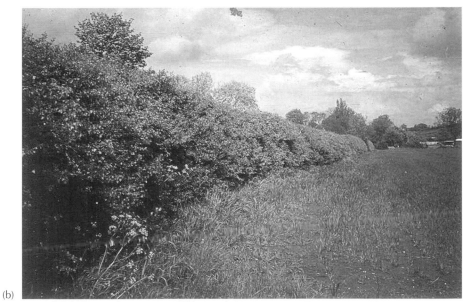

(b)

Fig. 6.14   A hedgerow can filter out downwind drift if it is sufficiently porous to avoid wind taking the spray up and over the hedge. Two examples of hedgerows (photographs from Silsoe Research Institute and GAM).

equipment. On the basis of these trials, a 50-m buffer zone was approved by the Environment Agency in the UK (Robinson *et al.*, 2000).

Studies of drift into woodland alongside a sprayed field (Fig. 6.15) indicated that penetration depended on the peripheral vegetation and to some extent wind speed, but where vegetation was low, spray droplets could penetrate 10 m, with the highest concentrations confined to within 5 m of the spray boom (Gove, 2004; Gove *et al.*, 2004). Needle-like foliage in windbreaks can capture two- to four-fold more spray than broad-leaved foliage (Ucar *et al.*, 2003). Thus, where 1% of applied herbicide drifts that far into woodland, the most sensitive plants can be adversely affected. Surveys of ancient woodland margins in Kent showed that species richness and abundance were least in margins alongside arable land compared to unimproved grassland (Gove, 2004).

Like crops, non-target vegetation will also vary in its susceptibility to herbicides. Most broad-leaved plants are to some extent susceptible to herbicides, which are used in cereals, such as wheat, to control broad-leaved weeds. Similarly, herbicides designed to control grass weeds will also adversely affect natural grass vegetation. With this variability, it has been suggested that the activity of new herbicides should be evaluated on six to ten species, including both mono- and dicotyledon species, in addition to crop species when assessing effects of pesticides on plants in terms of preserving biodiversity.

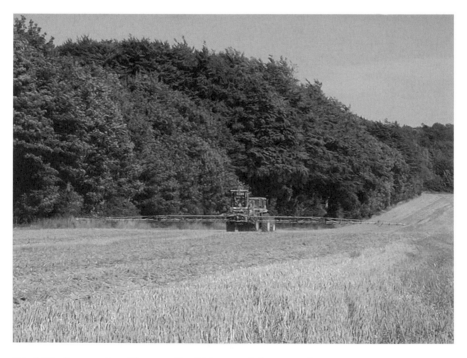

Fig. 6.15 Sprayer alongside a woodland (photograph from Benedict Gove).

Apart from effects on vegetation around treated fields, farmers must also be concerned with the possible effects of a persistent herbicide on any following crops, or whether a pesticide application will affect an adjacent crop, if inter-row or strip cropping is practised. By using a coarser spray to reduce airborne drift, there is always a possibility of increasing endo-drift, so the choice of pesticide and method of application do need to be considered carefully, where there is a greater diversity of crops.

Protecting birds

The Royal Society for the Protection of Birds has for many years been concerned at the decrease in a number of bird populations in the UK. The use of pesticides has been blamed, although it has also been recognised that many other changes in British agriculture have taken place over the past 50 years. The removal of hedgerows to allow more efficient use of large equipment is one of the most significant changes as it removed habitats suitable for many species. However, it is clear that pesticides can affect bird populations in several ways: first, direct effects due to poisoning; second, the ingestion of insects or vegetation that have been sprayed can have adverse effects; and third, the removal of vegetation can decrease populations of herbivorous insects that provide the food for certain bird species.

The overall effects of different pesticide types are shown in Table 6.2. Direct effects due to sprays are not expected unless a highly toxic insecticide is sprayed directly onto the birds. In Africa, certain weaver birds, *Quelea*, are known to destroy cereal crops ready for harvesting, so large colonies of these birds have been sprayed with the OP insecticide fenthion, when they

Table 6.2 Effects of different classes of pesticides on birds (adapted from Newton, 1998)

Pesticide type	Acute toxicity	Persistence	Bio-accumulation
Insecticides			
Natural pyrethrins	very low	low	very low
Organochlorine (e.g. DDT)	low	very high	very high
Cyclodienes	high	high	very high
Organophosphates	very high	low-moderate	low-moderate
Carbamates	very high	low-moderate	low-moderate
Pyrethroids	low-moderate	low	low
Insect growth regulators	very low	moderate	low
Fungicides			
Azole fungicides	low	low	low
Herbicides			
Chlorophenoxy herbicides	low	low	very low
Other (e.g. paraquat)	moderate	low	very low

congregated to roost at night. While this may save crops in fields in the immediate vicinity of the roost, it has never had any impact on the overall populations of this bird.

During the 1950s, treating cereal seeds with an organochlorine insecticide (e.g. dieldrin) to protect them from soil pests, including wheat bulb fly, led to the first bird mortalities, when hungry birds ate spring-sown seeds on or close to the soil surface. Rapid realisation of the cause of bird deaths led to the banning of sowing treated seed in the spring, when few other sources of seeds were readily available after the winter. Later, the consequence of predatory birds, such as the peregrine falcon, accumulating these persistent insecticides, became more evident with a rapid decline in their populations from 1955. Noting an abnormally high incidence of egg breakages in the falcon nest (eyries) led to the study of egg shell thickness (Radcliffe, 1967, 1970; Cooke, 1973). Overall insecticide residues in many species of birds that resulted in a reduction of egg thickness of about 17% or more was the cause of egg breakages occurring under natural conditions (Fig. 6.16; Table 6.3) (Newton, 1998). In North America, Hickey and Anderson (1968) were the first to report similar eggshell effects. Despite clear evidence of the adverse effect of organochlorine insecticides, 260,000 acres of wheat were aerially sprayed with endrin as late as 1981 in the USA, thereby contaminating many

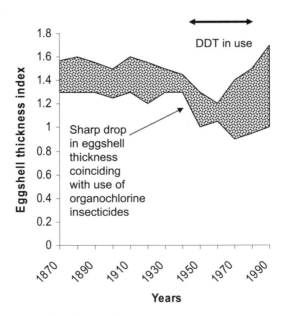

Fig. 6.16   Indication of shell-thickness index of British sparrowhawks, *Accipiter nisus*, from data collected at Monks Wood Research Station. Upper and lower indices are shown. Shell index measured as shell weight (mg)/shell length × breadth (mm). Shells became thinner abruptly after 1947 with the first widespread use of DDT and dieldrin; this was followed by recovery following restrictions on the pesticides' use (adapted from Newton, 1998).

Table 6.3 Comparison between plots with or without herbicide on weed, insect and game birds (from Newton, 1998)

	Herbicide-treated	No herbicide
Weeds		
Number per 0.25 m^2	2.1 ± 0.5	6.8 ± 1.0
Percentage weed cover	2.9 ± 0.6	14.2 ± 2.3
Insects		
As bird chick food-items per 0.5 m^2	18.9 ± 9.2	67.9 ± 23.4
Brood size		
Grey partridge	7.5 ± 0.8	10.0 ± 0.6
Pheasant	3.2 ± 0.5	6.9 ± 0.5

bird species with residues (Metcalf, 1984). Persistent organochlorines can still be detected in bird populations, for example in vultures in South Africa (van Wyk *et al.*, 2001) and in passerines in North America (Bartuszevige *et al.*, 2002). In Australia, a technique of flushing stomach contents of birds near or away from areas of insecticide use (cotton farms) was used to detect positive residues, including DDT and endosulfan, in 90% of the birds sampled (Sanchez-Bayo *et al.*, 1999).

Another research study examined why the number of grey partridge had declined so rapidly (Potts, 1986). Studies by the Game Conservancy showed that the application of herbicides was removing the weeds on which the survival of a number of insect species depended (Table 6.3). It was the lack of these insects that deprived the young partridge chicks of food during the early stages of their development. Thus, poor survival of the chicks resulted in the population crash. Farmers now can leave a strip around their fields, which is not treated with herbicides. This has developed into the concept of conservation headlands to foster partridges, pheasants and other game birds. Within the crop, regular use of herbicides – or indeed effective weed control by any means – will deprive herbivorous species of insects of their food source.

Studies on the yellowhammer (*Emberiza citrinella*) have examined the impact of insecticide sprays on chick survival (Morris *et al.*, 2005). As these birds also depend on an abundance of invertebrate food for chicks to develop, any insecticide spray at a critical stage during the breeding season will have an adverse effect on their foraging, and decrease populations. Numbers of invertebrates are generally higher in the hedge and field margins (Thomas and Marshall, 1999) (Table 6.4).

Several methods can be adopted to encourage bird populations on farms. In addition to conservation headlands, the use of no-spray buffer zones can be developed as 'set-aside' areas. However, these areas need to be managed, as uncared land will revert to woodland. Thus, in order to provide a better habitat for birds, these areas need to be sown with seeds of grasses and wild-

Table 6.4 Mean numbers of invertebrates in different positions of fields as indicated by suction samples (from Thomas and Marshall, 1999)

Position	Field A	Field B
Hedge	233.0	232.0
Sown field margin	155.8	147.8
Crop edge	84.5	58.3
Field	96.8	76.9

flowers to provide pollen, nectar and seeds suitable for the particular bird species that are to be encouraged in a given habitat. Wild flower mixtures will also encourage butterflies and bumble bees. Several agri-environmental projects are evaluating different approaches to habitat management. In Scotland, it was shown that up to 80 times as many birds were recorded where 'game' crops such as kale and black mustard were grown on set-aside, when compared with nearby conventional crops (Parish and Sotherton, 2004). In Japan, strips >300 m wide favoured bird diversity, whereas strips <50 m wide were unsuitable for feeding by egrets in irrigated rice areas, with some birds hardly occurring at field edges, indicating a need to consider both the width and location of strips (Maeda, 2005).

Protection of these areas requires careful thought about when and how pesticides are applied in the adjacent crop fields. The use of certain nozzles – for example, air-induction nozzles on the last downwind swath adjacent to a 'wildlife strip' – can significantly reduce drift into the area, but avoiding a pesticide spray at critical times of the year is also important, especially in relation to the breeding season of birds (Table 6.5). Thus, the application of certain insecticides and herbicides is better in the autumn on winter-sown cereals, rather than applying sprays in the spring and summer. Nevertheless, when farmers need to spray at these times, the impact on non-target species can be mitigated, if the least hazardous and more selective pesticide products are used to control specific insect pests or weeds. Where the location of specific weeds can be mapped, then patch spraying would also reduce the likelihood of adverse effects in the 'wildlife strip'.

Table 6.5 Guidelines of spraying in association with conservation headlands in the UK

Time of application	Autumn spraying	Spring spraying
Insecticides	Only by avoiding drift	Only prior to mid-March
Fungicides	Yes	Yes
Plant growth regulators	Yes	Yes
Herbicides		
Grass weeds	Only selective graminicides	Only selective graminicides
Broad-leaf weeds	No[*]	No[*]

[*]Some herbicides may be used if approved for a specific weed problem (e.g. *Galium aparine*).

Strips within crop fields, usually referred to as 'beetle banks', sown with tussock-forming grasses, such as red fescue and timothy grass, have also been advocated to conserve ground-dwelling carabid beetles, which are important aphid predators (Collins *et al.*, 2002). Studies have shown that the relatively high abundance and number of species of beetles within these field margins contribute significantly to invertebrate biodiversity in agricultural landscapes (Woodcock *et al.*, 2005).

The description above is related to the situation in the UK, where uptake of these environmentally friendly measures will depend on the response of farmers to the changes from the EU Common Agricultural Policy on subsidies for crops to payments for environmental stewardship. In parts of the world outside Europe there is also concern about environmental effects, and this has led so far to the banning of persistent organochlorine insecticides and other pesticides on the POP list. In the USA, the spray drift task force was set up to provide data for the EPA registration process.

Overall environmental impact assessments

Most registration authorities examine data on the impact of pesticides on specific key indicator species. The OECD has a project on pesticide terrestrial risk indictors and has published reports at www.oecd.org/env/pesticides. In the UK, the 'Pesticide Forum' publishes an annual report in which details of the various indicators of the impact of pesticides in the environment are described. There are various techniques which can be used to estimate the overall impact of pesticide use in the environment. In 2004, 17 indicators were used taking into account developments with the Voluntary Initiative. Using these indicators, the Forum is hoping to improve ways to measure the relationship between use, need and application rates to reduce environmental impact. Some pollution models rely on detailed knowledge of physical, chemical and microbial processes that affect the persistence and movement of pesticides in soil, air and water, and may not consider the effect of different organisms within an ecosystem. Some risk assessments consider the fate and exposure to pesticides and attempt to rank effects, while others consider different impacts over the lifetime of a product.

Margni *et al.* (2002) have advocated the need for a new quantified evaluation of the overall impact of pesticides on the health of humans and ecosystems. The proposed method considers different exposure effects (inhalation, intake via food and drinking water, etc.), transfers, such as soil to water and between water and air, as well as the fate of the pesticides and exposure to them. In developing their approach, these authors have assumed, for example, that following a field application of a water-based pesticide using a boom sprayer, 10% of the spray remains in the air (or returns to the air by volatilisation from foliar deposits). Furthermore, it was assumed that 85%

enters the soil and only 5% is retained on the crop. There are, then, dilution factors within the soil profile and transfer to surface waters. With subsequent analysis of residues in food (these are discussed more fully in Chapter 7), Margni *et al.* assume that following peeling, washing and processing of a food, the residue remaining is 5% of the tolerance value (i.e. the MRL). While these assumptions are not always appropriate, they develop characterisation factors that allow an estimate of the impact per kg of active ingredient. This then needs to be adjusted, depending on the amounts actually applied. Initial evaluation of the technique indicated that impacts on human health, the aquatic ecosystem and terrestrial ecosystem differed between the five fungicides examined. Also, in relation to human health, food intake resulted in the highest toxic exposure by 10^3-fold to 10^5-fold compared to drinking water or inhalation.

In the UK, pEMA is a computer-based decision support tool (Fig. 6.17) which estimates risks to a wide range of taxonomic groups in different environmental situations. Methods consistent with the UK regulatory assessments are used, but adjusted to take into account the formulation used and local conditions. Pathways along which the pesticide is dispersed in the environment are modelled to estimate concentrations in soil in the field and at its margin, in surface water and groundwater (Brown *et al.*, 2003). Predicted environmental concentrations (PECs) are then combined with toxicological data as toxicity:exposure ratios to facilitate risk assessments to be made. Combining the risk indices for individual applications of each active ingredient to form an aggregate score for a farm provided an index of the environmental performance or 'eco-rating' for the average field (Hart *et al.*, 2003). The p-EMA approach included the philosophy of integrated pest management, and was based on easily available farm data and an accessible database. Operator exposure and residues in crops were not included. Lewis *et al.* (2003) provide an overview of the system (Table 6.6), and how it compares with other indicators during the European Project CAPER (concerted action on pesticide risk indicators).

In this collaborative programme, the environmental risk of fifteen individual pesticide applications were compared using eight indicators (Table 6.7) (Reus *et al.*, 2002). It assumed that all pesticides, except glyphosate, were applied as foliar sprays to apple trees using an airblast sprayer. Pesticides included in the project were not necessarily approved in all the countries participating in the project. Surface water, groundwater and soil indicators gave similar rankings, but the overall score for the environment differed. Not unexpectedly, a ranking based on 'kilograms of active ingredient' was not correlated with rankings by risk indicators.

Another composite scoring index (EcoRR; the ecological relative index) has been developed in Australia (Sanchez-Bayo *et al.*, 2002), and has been evaluated in the context of 37 pesticides that can be used in a cotton development.

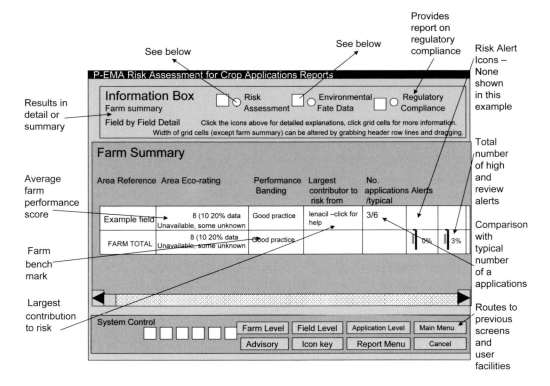

Field by Field – Risk data

Example field

Pesticide active applied	Eco-rating Mammals	Eco-rating Birds	Eco-rating Earthworms	Eco-rating Algae
thiram	-45	-44	0	0
lenacil	0	-15	0	-51
carbendazim	0	0	-27	0
flusilazole	-35	-18	0	0
Mean Eco-rating	-20	-19	-6	-12

Field by Field – Fate Data

Example field Pesticide active Substance	Effective application [a.s.] rate [g.ha]	Annual groundwater conc [ug/l]	Accum. Conc. in field: soil [mg/kg]	Accum.conc in margin soil[mg.kg]
thiram	8.30	0 000 [60%]	0.0111 [100%]	0 0000 [100%]
lanacil	176.00	0 019 [70%]	0.2347 [100%]	0 0065 [100%]
carbendazim	16.43	0 000 [100%]	0.0219 [100%]	0.0030 [100%]
fusilazole	32.85	0 000 [80%]	0.0438 [100%]	0.0060 [100%]

Fig. 6.17 Communicating risk information to the user (courtesy of Kathy Lewis). Selection of a specific 'Information Box' on the computer screen provides additional data as illustrated above for Risk data and Fate data.

Table 6.6   EMA Eco-scores and relative rankings of pesticides used to control aphids and thus virus yellows in sugar beet (from Lewis *et al.*, 2003)

Pesticide	Mammals	Birds	Earthworms	Average aquatics	Honey bees	Ground water	Overall
			Eco-score (with relative ranking in bold)				
Aldicarb	−71 **1**	−100 **1**	no data	−0 **4**	0 **4**	−68 **1**	−45 **1**
Deltamethrin	−28 **3**	0 **4**	0 **2**	−58 **2**	−33 **2**	0 **2**	−20 **4**
Pirimicarb	−58 **2**	−83 **2**	−25 **1**	−35 **3**	−17 **3**	0 **2**	−36 **2**
Imidacloprid	−7 **5**	−35 **3**	0 **2**	0 **4**	0 **4**	0 **2**	−13 **5**
Lambacyhalothrin	−27 **4**	0 **4**	0 **2**	−60 **1**	−37 **1**	0 **2**	−21 **3**

Note: Aldicarb applied as granules, and imidacloprid as a seed treatment; others applied as foliar sprays. Rating **1** is worst case, **5** is best case.

Table 6.7   Pesticide risk indicators evaluated in the CAPER project (from Reus *et al.*, 2002)

Number	Risk indicator	Acronym	Country
1	Environmental yardstick	EYP	The Netherlands
2	HD	HD	Denmark
3	SYNOPS-2	SYNOPS-2	Germany
4	Environmental performance indicator of pesticides	p-EMA	UK
5	Pesticide environmental impact indicator	Ipest	France
6	Environmental potential risk	EPRIP	Italy
7	System for protecting the environmental impact of pesticides	SyPEP	Belgium
8	Pesticide environmental risk indicator	PERI	Sweden

It was considered that the EcoRR score reflected the potential risk to eco-systems, as it takes account of biodiversity, yet is less dependent on toxicity to sensitive species.

Another approach proposed by Padovani *et al.* (2004) is an environmental potential risk indictor for pesticides (EPRIP), which is based on the ratio of PEC estimated at local level with short-term toxicity data. It reflects a worse case scenario, but can identify those crops on which pesticide use presents the highest risk to non-target organisms. It does this by taking account of multiple applications, synergistic effects and different formulation types. Thus, users can assess different management options.

When these environmental risk assessments are carried out on farms, many other factors must also be taken into consideration. In assessing the five insecticides shown in Table 6.6, aldicarb granules and imidacloprid seed treatment are prophylactic treatments in areas where the risk of virus yellows infection is high. Aldicarb would be preferred, if there is also a nematode problem. However, the sugar industry in the UK has an early warning system for aphids (Dewar, 1994), so a spray may only be required if and when an aphid infestation occurs. Pirimicarb is the most selective foliar spray and ideal for aphids, but the farmer may wish to use a pyrethroid insecticide for greater persistence and a broader spectrum of activity. Costs will also be an important consideration. Thus, in each crop and agroecosystem, local knowledge is important as well as the overall assessment of ecological impact. Various tools have been developed to assist decision making on farms, for example whether a herbicide can be used (Fig. 6.18).

Locust control until 1985 had relied on use of dieldrin, which was stockpiled in various African countries. Following the banning of this insecticide, there was a major problem of disposal of the large stocks of obsolete pesticides. The FAO set up a programme to cope with this, but in anticipation of further locust plagues a small group was established to advise on suitable insecticides for locust control. The advisory group listed a number of active ingredients that had been shown to be effective in field trials, and then also provided assessments of environment impact on selected non-target organisms (Tables 6.8 and 6.9) (Anon, 2005). This allowed users a choice between

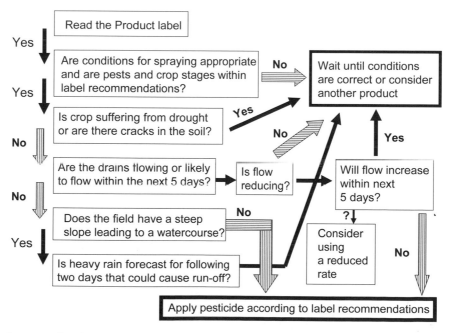

Fig. 6.18 Flow diagram regarding the decision on whether to spray a particular herbicide, depending on soil and rainfall (adapted from Voluntary Initiative webpage).

Table 6.8 Risk to non-target organisms at verified dose rates against the desert locust. Risk is classified as low (L), medium (M) or high (H). See Table 6.9 for the classification criteria

Insecticide	Aquatic organisms		Terrestrial vertebrates			Terrestrial non-target arthropods		
	Fish	Arthropods	Mammals	Birds	Reptiles	Bees	Antagonists	Soil insects
Bendiocarb	M[2]	L[3]	M[1]	L[3]	–	H[1]	H[3]	M[3]
Chlorpyrifos	M[3]	H[2]	L[3]	M[3]	M[3]	H[1]	H[3]	–
Deltamethrin	L[3]	H[3]	L[3]	L[3]	L[3]	M[1]	M[3]	M[3]
Diflubenzuron (blanket)	L[3]	H[3]	L[1]	L[1]	–	L[1]†	M[2]	M[3]
Diflubenzuron (barrier)*	L	(H)	L	L	–	L†	L[3]	(M)
Fenitrothion	L[3]	M[3]	L[3]	M[3]	M[3]	H[1]	H[3]	H[3]
Fipronil (barrier)*	L[3]	M[3]	L[3]	L[3]	M[3]	(H)	H[3]	H[3]
Lambda-cyhalothrin	L[2]	H[2]	L[1]	L[1]	–	M[1]	M[3]	H[3]
Malathion	L[2]	M[2]	L[3]	L[3]	–	H[3]	H[3]	H[3]
Metarhizium anisopliae (IMI 330189)	L[2]	L[2]	L[1]	L[1]	L[2]	L[3]	L[3]	L[3]
Teflubenzuron (blanket)	L[1]	H[2]	L[1]	L[1]	–	L[1]‡	M[1]	–
Triflumuron (blanket)	L[1]	H[2]	L[1]	L[1]	L[3]	L[1]‡	L[3]	L[3]
Triflumuron (barrier) *	L	(H)	L	L	L[3]	L[1]‡	L[3]	L[3]

The index next to the classification describes the level of availability of data:

[1] Classification based on laboratory and registration data with species which do not occur in locust areas.

[2] Classification based on laboratory data or small-scale field trials with indigenous species from locust areas.

[3] Classification based on medium- to large-scale field trials and operational data from locust areas (mainly desert locust, but also migratory and brown locust).

* If no field data are available, the risk of barrier treatments is extrapolated from blanket treatments. However, it is expected to be considerably lower if at least 50% of the area remains uncontaminated for a period long enough to allow recovery of affected fauna, and if barriers are not sprayed over surface water. Risk classes are therefore shown in brackets unless the blanket treatment was already considered to pose low risk, and no reference is made to the level of data availability. More field data are needed to confirm that products posing a medium or high risk as blanket sprays can be downgraded to 'L' when applied as barrier sprays.

† At normal use, diflubenzuron is not harmful to the brood of honey bee.

‡ Benzoylureas are safe to adult worker bees, but some may cause damage to the brood of exposed colonies.

(–): insufficient data.

Table 6.9 Criteria applied for the environmental risk classification used in Table 6.8. See text for further explanations

A. Laboratory toxicity data

Group	Parameter	Risk class low (L)	Risk class medium (M)	Risk class high (H)	Reference
Fish	risk ratio (PEC[1]/LC$_{50}$[2])	<1	1–10	>10	FAO/ Locustox[4]
Aquatic arthropods	risk ratio (PEC/LC$_{50}$)	<1	1–10	>10	FAO/ Locustox
Reptiles, birds, mammals	risk ratio (PEC/LD$_{50}$[3])	<0.01	0.01–0.1	0.1	EPPO[5]
Bees	risk ratio (recommended dose rate/LD$_{50}$)	<50	50–500	>500	PRG[6]/ EPPO[7]
Other terrestrial arthropods	acute toxicity (%) at recommended dose rate	<50%	50–99%	>99%	IOBC[8]

B. Field data (well conducted field trials and control operations)

Group	Parameter	Risk class low (L)	Risk class medium (M)	Risk class high (H)	Reference
Fish	evidence of mortality	none	incidental	massive	PRG
Aquatic arthropods	population reduction	<50%	50–90%	>90%	PRG
Reptiles, birds, mammals	evidence of mortality	none	incidental	massive	PRG
Bees	evidence of mortality	not significant	incidental	massive	EPPO
Other terrestrial arthropods	population reduction	<25%	25–75%	>75%	IOBC

[1]PEC: Predicted Environmental Concentration after treatment at the recommended dose rate.
[2]LC$_{50}$: median lethal concentration.
[3]LD$_{50}$: median lethal dose.
[4]FAO/Locustox: FAO Locustox project in Senegal (Everts *et al.*, 1997, 1998).
[5]EPPO: European and Mediterranean Plant Protection Organization (EPPO, 2003a).
[6]PRG: Pesticide Referee Group.
[7]EPPO (2003b).
[8]International Organization for Biological and Integrated Control of Noxious Animals and Plants (Hassan, 1994).
Note: As a result of a greater error associated with population estimates of terrestrial arthropods, the lower limits of the different risk classes are lower than for aquatic arthropods.

the quick-acting organophosphates and pyrethroids for rapid control of locusts in swarms, while being able to use either more selective chitin inhibitors against nymphs or a broad-spectrum insecticide used at low dose as a barrier treatment. In areas of extreme ecological sensitivity, a biopesticide based on *Metarhizium* was recommended. However, the greatest task in locust control is to be able to forecast when an upsurge could develop and to deploy sufficient resources to control hoppers and incipient swarms rapidly to prevent swarms developing and migrating. The 2003 upsurge was predicted, and in October 2003 the FAO issued an alert. However, funds and resources in West Africa were not forthcoming in sufficient time to stop the upsurge occurring and initially causing crop damage in Mauritania. In contrast, in the Sudan and Saudi Arabia, similar indications of an upsurge were controlled rapidly. The setting up of the Emergency Programme EMPRES to operate in the countries around the Red Sea was one factor that enabled the rapid response. Clearly, the more rapidly a potential upsurge can be controlled the less insecticide will be needed. By acting earlier against hoppers, the insect growth regulators and barrier treatments are also likely to reduce environmental impact. The slower-acting biopesticide would also be appropriate in situations where crops were not yet at risk.

This chapter has shown that the authorities have responded to problems encountered when pesticides cause unacceptable adverse effects in the environment. The requirements for registration now demand far more environmental data, and great care is taken to examine all aspects of potential problems. Inevitably, some chemicals have been registered as subsequent adverse effects were not foreseen. DDT is a good example of a very effective insecticide of low mammalian toxicity, but its effects on birds and the food chain had not been realised when it was initially promoted. As our knowledge base continues to expand, conditions for registration have become more precise.

References

Anon (2001) *Groundwater Protection Code: Use and disposal of sheep dip compounds*. DEFRA, UK.

Anon (2005) *Report of the Locust Pesticide Referee Group*. 8th Meeting, FAO, Rome.

Armbrust, K.L. and Peeler, H.B. (2002) Effects of formulation on the run-off of imidacloprid from turf. *Pest Management Science* **58**, 702–706.

Arnold, G.L., Luckenbach, M.W. and Unger, M.A. (2004) Runoff from tomato cultivation in the estuarine environment: Biological effects of farm management practices. *Journal of Experimental Marine Biology and Ecology* **298**, 323–346.

Barraclough, D., Kearney, T. and Croxford, A. (2005) Bound residues: Environmental solution or future problem? *Environmental Pollution* **133**, 85–90.

Bartuszevige, A.M., Capparella, A.P., Harper, R.G., Frick, J.A., Criley, B., Doty, K. and Erhart, E. (2002) Organochlorine pesticide contamination in grassland-nesting passerines that breed in North America. *Environmental Pollution* **117**, 225–232.

Berenzen, N., Kumke, T., Schultz, H.K. and Schultz, R. (2005a) Macroinvertebrate community structure in agricultural streams: Impact of runoff-related pesticide contamination. *Ecotoxicology and Environmental Safety* **70**, 37–46.

Berenzen, N., Lentzen-Godding, A., Probst, M., Schultz, H., Schultz, R. and Liess M. (2005b) A comparison of predicted and measured levels of runoff-related pesticide concentrations in small lowland streams on a landscape level. *Chemosphere* **58**, 683–691.

Blanchoud, H., Farrugia, F. and Mouchel, J.M. (2004) Pesticide uses and transfer in urbanised catchments. *Chemosphere* **55**, 905–913.

Brown, C.D., Bellamy, P.H. and Dubus, I.G. (2002) Prediction of pesticide concentrations found in rivers in the UK. *Pest Management Science* **58**, 363–373.

Brown, C.D., Hart, A., Lewis, K.A. and Dubus, I.G. (2003) p-EMA (I): Simulating the environmental fate of pesticides for a farm-level risk assessment system. *Agronomie* **23**, 67–74.

Brown, C.D., Dubus, I.G., Fogg, P., Spirlet, M. and Gustin, C. (2004a) Exposure to sulfosulfuron in agricultural drainage ditches: Field monitoring and scenario-based modelling. *Pest Management Science* **60**, 765–776.

Brown, R.B., Carter, M.H. and Stephenson, G.R. (2004b) Buffer zone and windbreak effects on spray deposition in a simulated wetland. *Pest Management Science* **60**, 1085–1090.

Butler-Ellis, C. and Bradley, A. (2002) The influence of formulation on spray drift. *Aspects of Applied Biology* **66**, 251–258.

Cagauan, A.G. (1995) The impact of pesticides on ricefield vertebrates with emphasis on fish. In: Pingali, P.L. and Roger, P.A. (eds.), *Impact of Pesticides on Farmer Health and the Rice Environment*. Kluwer, Dordrecht, pp. 203–248.

Collins, K.L., Boatman, N.D., Wilcox, A. Holland, J.M. and Chaney, K. (2002) Influence of beetle banks on cereal aphid predation in winter wheat. *Agriculture, Ecosystems and Environment* **93**, 337–350.

Cooke, A.S. (1973) Shell thinning in avian eggs by environmental pollutants. *Environmental Pollution* **4**, 85–152.

Crane, M., Whitehouse, P., Comber, S., Watts, C., Giddings, J., Moore, D.R.J. and Grist, E. (2003) Evaluation of probabilistic risk assessment in the UK: Chlorpyrifos use on top fruit. *Pest Management Science* **59**, 512–526.

Cross, J.V., Murray, R.A., Walklate, P.J. and Richardson, G.M. (2004) Pesticide dose Adjustment to the Crop Environment (PACE): Efficacy evaluations in UK apple orchards 2002–2003. *Aspects of Applied Biology* **71**, 287–294.

Dabrowski, J.M., Bollen, A., Bennett, E.R. and Schulz, R. (2005) Pesticide interception by emergent aquatic macrophytes: Potential to mitigate spray-drift input in agricultural streams. *Agriculture, Ecosystems and Environment* **111**, 340–348.

Davis, B.N., Brown, M.J. and Frost, A.J. (1993) Selection of receptors for measuring spray drift deposition and comparison with bioassays with special reference to the shelter effect of hedges. *Brighton Crop Protection Conference – Weeds*, pp. 139–144.

Davis, B.N., Frost, A.J. and Yates, T.J. (1994a) Bioassays of insecticide drift from air assisted sprayers in an apple orchard. *Journal of Horticultural Science* **69**, 703–708.

Davis, B.N., Brown, M.J., Frost, A.J., Yates, T.J. and Plant, R.A. (1994b) The effects of hedges on spray deposition and on the biological impact of pesticide spray drift. *Ecotoxicology and Environmental Safety* **27**, 281–293.

De Snoo, G.R. (1999) Unsprayed field margins: Effects on environment, biodiversity and agricultural practice. *Landscape and Urban Planning* **46**, 151–160.

De Snoo, G.R. and de Witt, P.J. (1998) Buffer zones for reducing pesticide drift to ditches and risks to aquatic organisms. *Ecotoxicology and Environmental Safety* **41**, 112–118.

De Snoo, G.R. and van der Poll, R.J. (1999) Effect of herbicide drift on adjacent boundary vegetation. *Agriculture, Ecosystems and Environment* **73**, 1–6.

Dewar, A.M. (1994) The virus yellows warning scheme – an integrated pest management system for beet in the UK. In: Leather, S.R., Watt, A.D., Mills, N.J. and

Walters, K.F.A. (eds.), *Individuals, Populations, and Patterns in Ecology.* Atheneum Press, Newcastle on Tyne, pp. 173–185.

Douthwaite, R.J. and Tingle, C.C.D. (1994) *DDT in the Tropics: The impact on wildlife in Zimbabwe of ground-spraying for tsetse fly control.* Natural Resources Institute, Chatham.

Elliott, J.G. and Wilson, B.J. (1983) The influence of weather on the efficiency and safety of pesticide application: the drift of herbicides. *British Crop Protection Council Occasional publication No. 3.*

EPPO/Council of Europe (2003a) Environmental risk assessment scheme of plant protection products – Chapter 10: Honeybees. *OEPP/EPPO Bulletin* **33**, 141–145.

EPPO/Council of Europe (2003b) Environmental risk assessment scheme of plant protection products – Chapter 11: Terrestrial vertebrates. *OEPP/EPPO Bulletin* **33**, 211–238.

Everts, J.W., Mbaye, D. and Barry, O. (Eds.) (1997) *Environmental Side-effects of Locust and Grasshopper Control.* Vol. 1. FAO: GCP/SEN/053/NET. Rome, Dakar.

Everts, J.W., Mbaye, D., Barry, O. and Mullié, W. (Eds.) (1998) *Environmental Side-effects of Locust and Grasshopper Control.* Vols. 2 and 3. FAO: GCP/SEN/053/NET. Rome, Dakar.

Farooq, M., Balachandar, R., Wulfson, D. and Wolf, T.M. (2001) Agricultural sprays in cross-flow and drift. *Journal of Agricultural Engineering Research* **78**, 347–358.

Fox, P.J. and Matthiessen, P. (1982) Acute toxicity to fish of low-dose aerosol applications in relation to control tsetse fly in the Okavango Delta, Botswana. *Environmental Pollution Ser A* **27**, 129–142.

Ganzelmeier, R. and Rautmann, D. (2000) Drift, drift reducing sprayers and sprayer testing. *Aspects of Applied Biology* **57**, 1–10.

Ganzelmeier, H. (2005) GIS-based application of plant protection products – Examples from research and application. Paper presented at the Conference on Environmentally Friendly Spray Application Techniques, Warsaw (PL), October 2004. *Annual Review of Agricultural Engineering* **4**(1), 245–255.

Ganzelmeier, R., Rautmann, D., Spangenberg, R., Streloke, M., Herrmann, M., Wenzelburger, H.J. and Walter, H.F. (1995) *Studies on the Spray Drift of Plant Protection Products.* 111pp, BBA, Germany.

Gilbert, A.J. (2000) Local environmental risk assessment for pesticides. *Aspects of Applied Biology* **57**, 83–90.

Gove, B. (2004) *The impact of pesticide spray drift and fertilizer over-spread on the ground flora of ancient woodland.* PhD. Thesis, University of London.

Gove, B., Ghazoury, J., Power, S. and Buckley, P. (2004) *The Impacts of Pesticide Spray Drift and Fertiliser Over-spread on the Ground Flora of Ancient Woodland.* English Nature Research Reports, 614.

Grant, I.F. and Tingle, C.D. (2002) *Ecological Monitoring Methods Handbook.* Natural Resources Institute, University of Greenwich.

Hart, A., Brown, C.D., Lewis, K.A. and Tzilivakis, J. (2003) p-EMA (II): Evaluating ecological risks of pesticides for farm-level risk assessment system. *Agronomie* **23**, 75–84.

Hassan, S.A. (1994) Activities of the IOBC/WPRS working group 'Pesticides and Beneficial Organisms'. *IOBC/WPRS Bulletin* **17**(10), 1–5.

Herbst, A. (2003) *Pesticide Formulation and Drift Potential.* The BCPC International Congress, pp. 255–260.

Hewitt, A.J. (2000) Spray drift modelling, labelling and management in the US. *Aspects of Applied Biology* **57**, 11–19.

Hickey, J.J. and Anderson, D.W. (1968) Chlorinated hydrocarbons and eggshell changes in raptorial and fish-eating birds. *Science NY* **162**, 271–273.

Koch, H. and Weisser, P. (2004) A proposal for a higher tier investigation of pesticide drift exposure to non-target organisms (NTO) in field trials. *Nachrichtenbl. Deut. Pflanzenschutzd.* **56**, S180–S183.

Koch, H., Strub, O. and Weisser, P. (2004a) The patchiness of pesticide drift deposition patterns in plant canopies. *Nachrichtenbl. Deut. Pflanzenschutzd.* **56**, S25–S29.

Koch, H., Weisser, P. and Strub, O. (2004b) Comparison of dose response of pesticide spray deposits versus drift deposits. *Nachrichtenbl. Deut. Pflanzenschutzd.* **56**, S30–S34.

Lane, A.G. and Butler-Ellis, C. (2003) Assessment of environmental concentrations of pesticide from spray drift. *The BCPC International Congress*, pp. 501–506.

Lewis, K.A., Brown, C.D., Hart, A. and Tzilivakis, J. (2003) p-EMA (III): Overview and application of a software system designed to assess environmental risk of agricultural pesticides. *Agronomie* **23**, 85–96.

Maeda, T. (2005) Bird use of rice field strips of varying width in the Kanto Plain of central Japan. *Agriculture, Ecosystems and Environment* **105**, 347–351.

Margni, M., Rossier, D., Crettaz, P. and Jolliet, O. (2002) Life cycle impact assessment of pesticides on human health and ecosystems. *Agriculture, Ecosystems and Environment* **93**, 379–392.

Metcalf, R.L. (1984) An increasing public concern. *EPA Journal* **10**, 30–31. (Also in Pimental, D. and Lehman, H. (eds.) (1993) *The Pesticide Question.* Chapman & Hall, New York.)

Miller, D.R. and Stoughton, T.E. (2000) Response of spray drift from aerial applications at forest edge to atmospheric stability. *Agricultural and Forestry Meteorology* **100**, 49–58.

Morris, A.J., Wilson, J.D., Whittingham, M.J. and Bradbury, R. (2005) Indirect effects of pesticides on breeding yellowhammer (*Emberiza citrinella*). *Agriculture, Ecosystems and Environment* **106**, 1–16.

Muller, K., Deurer, M., Hartmann, H., Bach, M., Spiteller, M. and Frede, H.-G. (2003) Hydrological characterisation of pesticide loads using hydrograph separation at different scales in a German catchment. *Journal of Hydrology* **273**, 1–17.

Nakano, Y., Miyazaki, A., Yoshida, T., Ono, K. and Inoue, T. (2004) A study on pesticide runoff in the Kozakura River, Japan. *Water Research* **38**, 3017–3022.

Neumann, M., Schulz, R., Schäfer, K., Müller, W., Mannheller, W. and Liess, M. (2002) The significance of entry routes as point and non-point sources of pesticides in small streams. *Water Research* **36**, 835–842.

Newton, I. (1998) *Population Limitation in Birds.* Academic Press, San Diego.

Padovani, L., Trevisan, M. and Capri, E. (2004) A calculation procedure to assess potential environmental risk of pesticides at the farm level. *Ecological Indicators* **4**, 111–123.

Parish, D.M.B. and Sotherton, N.W. (2004) Game crops as summer habitat for farmland songbirds in Scotland. *Agriculture Ecosystems and Environment* **104**, 429–438.

Parkin, C.S., Walklate, P.J. and Nicholls, J.W. (2003) Effect of drop evaporation on spray drift and buffer zone risk assessments. *The BCPC International Congress*, pp. 261–266.

Planas, S., Solanelles, F. and Fillat, A. (2002) Assessment of recycling tunnel sprayers in Mediterranean vineyards and apple orchards. *Biosystems Engineering* **82**, 45–52.

Potts, G.R. (1986) *The Partridge: Pesticides, predation and conservation.* Collins, London.

Radcliffe, D.A. (1967) Decrease in eggshell weight in certain birds of prey. *Nature (London)* **215**, 208–210.

Radcliffe, D.A. (1970) Changes attributable to pesticides in egg breakage frequency and egg shell thickness in some British birds. *Journal of Applied Ecology* **7**, 67–115.

Ramwell, C.T., Heather, A.I.J. and Shepherd, A.J. (2002) Herbicide loss following application to a roadside. *Pest Management Science* **58**, 695–701.

Ramwell, C.T., Heather, A.I.J. and Shepherd, A.J. (2004) Herbicide loss following application to a railway. *Pest Management Science* **60**, 556–564.

Rasmussen, L.H., Kroghsbo, S., Frisvad, J.C. and Hansen, H.C.B. (2003) Occurrence of the carcinogenic bracken constituent ptaquiloside in fronds, topsoils and organic soil layers in Denmark. *Chemosphere* **51**, 117–127.

Reus, J., Leendertse, P., Bockstaller, C., Fomsgaard, I., Gutsche, V., Lewis, K., Nilsson, C., Pussemier, L., Trevisa, M., van der Werf, H., Alfarroba, F., Blumel, S., Isart, J., McGath, D. and Seppala, T. (2002) Comparison and evaluation of eight pesticide environmental risk indicators developed in Europe and recommendations for future use. *Agriculture, Ecosystems and Environment* **90**, 177–187.

Robinson, R.C., Parsons, R.G., Barbe, G., Patel, P.T. and Murphy, S. (2000) Drift control and buffer zones for helicopter spraying of bracken (*Pteridium aquilinum*). *Agriculture, Ecosystems and Environment* **79**, 215–231.

Ropke, B., Bach, M. and Frede, H.-G. (2004) DRIPS – a DSS for estimating the input quantity of pesticides for German river basins. *Environmental Modelling and Software* **19**, 1021–1028.

Sanchez-Bayo, F., Ward, R. and Beasley, H. (1999) A new technique to measure bird's dietary exposure to pesticides. *Analytica Chimica Acta* **399**, 173–183.

Sanchez-Bayo, F., Baskaran, S. and Kennedy, I.R. (2002) Ecological relative risk (EcoRR): Another approach for risk assessment of pesticides in agriculture. *Agriculture, Ecosystems and Environment* **91**, 37–57.

Sankararamakrishnan, N., Sharma, A.K. and Sanghi, R. (2004) Organochlorine and organophosphorus pesticide residues in ground water and surface waters of Kanpur, Uttar Pradesh, India. *Environmental International* **31**, 113–120.

Schultz, R. (2001) Rainfall-induced sediment and pesticide input from orchards into the Lourens river, Western Cape South Africa: Importance of a single event. *Water Research* **35**, 1869–1876.

Sidahmed, M.M., Awadalla, H.H. and Haidar, M.A. (2004) Symmetrical multi-foil shields for reducing spray drift. *Biosystems Engineering* **88**, 305–312.

Skark, C., Zullei-Seibert N., Willme, U., Gatzemann, U. and Schlett, C. (2004) Contribution of non-agricultural pesticides to pesticide load in surface water. *Pest Management Science* **60**, 525–530.

Southcombe, E.S.E., Miller, P.C.H., Ganzelmeier, H., Miralles, A. and Hewitt, A.J. (1997) The international (BCPC) spray classification system including a drift potential factor. *Proc Brighton Crop Protection Conference*, pp. 371–380.

Tariq, M.I., Afzal, S. and Hussain, I. (2003) Pesticides in shallow groundwater of Bahawalnagar, Muzafargarth, D.G. Khan and Rajan Pur districts of Punjab, Pakistan. *Environmental International* **30**, 471–479.

Thomas, M.B. and Marshall, E.J.P. (1999) Arthropod abundance and diversity in different vegetated margins of arable fields. *Agriculture, Ecosystems and Environment* **72**, 131–144.

Ucar, T., Hall, F.R., Tew, J.E. and Hacker, J.K. (2003) Wind tunnel studies on spray deposition on leaves of tree species used in windbreaks and exposure to bees. *Pest Management Science* **59**, 358–364.

Van Wyk, E., Bouwman, H., van der Bank, H., Verdoorn, G.H. and Hofmann, D. (2001) Persistent organochlorine pesticides detected in blood and tissue samples of vultures from different localities in South Africa. *Comparative Biochemistry and Physiology Part C* **129**, 243–264.

Woodcock, B.A., Westbury, D.B., Potts, S.G., Harris, S.J. and Brown, V.K. (2005) Establishing field margins to promote beetle conservation in arable farms. *Agriculture, Ecosystems and Environment* **107**, 255–266.

7 Residues in food

The foliar application of a pesticide to a crop is a very inefficient process, with only a fraction of the pesticide actually being retained on plants and some being lost to the ground. The amount retained on the crop depends on many factors, including the formulation of pesticide used, the volume of spray applied, the type of equipment used (e.g. with air assistance) and the quality of the spray (e.g. the droplet sizes). The physical characteristics of the foliage – especially the leaf surface – will also determine whether droplets bounce off the leaves or are retained. When the volume of spray liquid applied was high (>500 l/ha), only about 20% of the pesticide was deposited on the crop, with most of the chemical being wasted on the soil. (Fig. 7.1). The trend has been to reduce the spray volume, and many sprays are now applied at less than 150 l/ha, so increasing spray efficiency, although as mentioned previously, if the droplet size is too large then more pesticide is likely to be deposited on the soil.

The droplets that remain on the surface of the plant will dry and form a deposit. From this deposit, the active ingredient will either stay on the surface to control pests that walk or land on the outside of the plant, penetrate through the outer surface of the plant, or be lost from the surface. The latter effect may be caused by rain, especially if it occurs with an hour or so of the pesticide being applied, or the pesticide may volatilise from the surface or be abraded physically by other surfaces. Further losses occur as the active ingredient is degraded either within the plant or on the surface, for example by ultraviolet light. The concern in terms of residues in crops is the amount of active ingredient that remains on or within the harvested product.

A maximum residue level (MRL) is derived from field trials carried out according to good agricultural practice (GAP), including the observance of a pre-harvest interval (PHI; the period between the last application and harvesting) to determine the highest legally permitted residue concentration that could be present in a crop. The intention is that there will be a legally enforceable limit to check whether farmers do follow GAP. The MRL is not based on the acceptable daily intake (ADI) of a pesticide residue but is usually derived from data obtained from eight to sixteen field trials (Hyder and Travis, 2003), but as the agrochemical companies concentrate on major crops, in many situations the MRL is set at the limit of detection. In order to minimise the residue, farmers have to follow advice and ensure that the PHI is observed. When a crop has to be treated on several occasions and is harvested over a long period, it is more difficult to check that the interval is

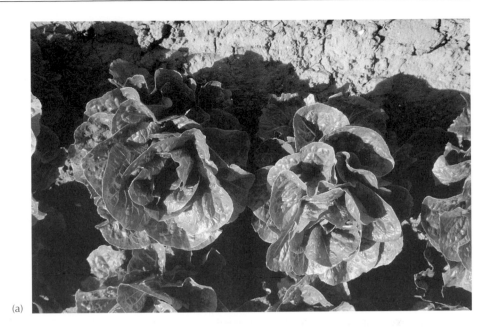

(a)

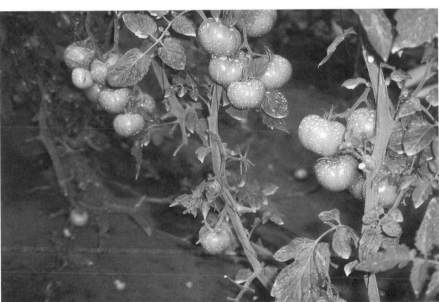

(b)

Fig. 7.1 Excessive spray deposits on (a) lettuce and (b) tomato crops (photographs GAM).

fully effective. In these situations, pesticides with a known short persistence are preferable to chemicals such as the organochlorine insecticides, most of which have been withdrawn from use as they are highly persistent.

A check on the residue level in a crop is made by sampling them to determine whether they contain any detectable residues (Figs. 7.2–7.4).

Official data obtained from these samples are analysed by the Government Pesticide Residue Committee, and are published. The results indicate how many samples have no detectable residue and, from those containing residues, whether the amount of the active ingredient exceeds the MRL at, or shortly after, harvest. Residue data are also obtained from processed food (e.g. bread) or on commodities not grown in the country, but imported (e.g. bananas). As an example, during 2001, among 4003 samples analysed for a wide range of pesticides, no detectable residues were found in 71% of cases. Residues below the MRL were found in 28% of samples, and only 0.7% had a higher residue or contained a pesticide not approved in the UK. Data from a selection of crops showing the number of samples analysed for certain crops in recent years are given in Table 7.1.

Data for 2003 showed that out of 4071 samples only 27 (0.7%) had a residue exceeding the MRL and 75% had no detectable residue of the pesticides sought. Nevertheless, media coverage always paints a more alarming picture, such as '93% of the (non-organic) oranges that you buy have residues', and '78% of apples', without any indication of which residues were present or that the presence of small residues is not a health concern.

Up-to-date information relevant to the UK is available at www.pesticides. gov.uk by examining the PRC (Pesticides Residues Committee) reports. Other information on MRLs and what pesticides may be used can be obtained by subscribing to the Central Science Laboratory database 'Liaison', which is an on-line knowledge system that allows rapid identification of approved

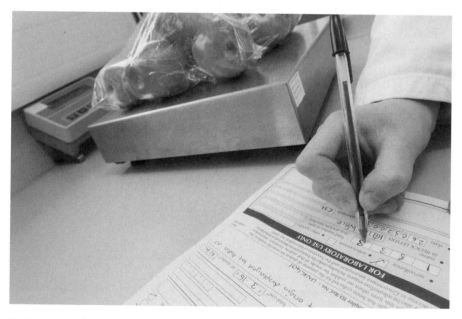

Fig. 7.2 Recording details of samples for residue analysis (CSL Photograph).

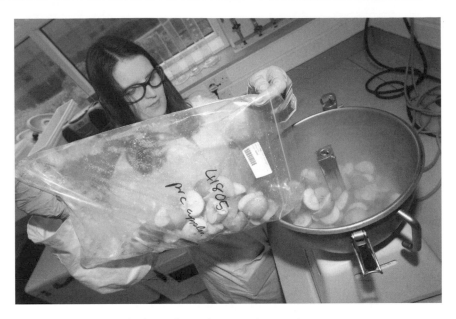

Fig. 7.3   Processing samples for residue analysis (CSL Photograph).

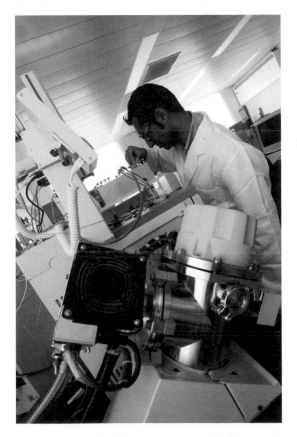

Fig. 7.4   Analysis of sample extracts by gas chromatography (CSL Photograph).

Table 7.1 Pesticide residues detected between 1991 and 2002 for selected crops in the UK as reported by the Pesticides Residues Committee (adapted from Foster *et al.*, 2003)

Crop	No. of samples tested	% with residues	%>MRL	No. of pesticides found
Apple	396	44	0	25
Banana	181	65	2.8	7
Carrot	369	64	0.8	12
Celery	276	66	4.0	30
Grapes	382	44	2.1	46
Lettuce	803	58	3.7	37
Mushroom	255	11	0.8	5
Onion	146	48	0	1
Orange	303	95	2.0	30
Potato	1722	37	0.3	15
Strawberry	383	67	0.3	12
Tomato	359	23	0.3	26

uses of pesticides in the UK. With the latest techniques in analytical chemistry, it is now possible to detect and measure extremely small quantities of a pesticide within a large sample of the commodity (e.g. parts per billion). A residue below the level of detection is sometimes assumed to be just below the limit of quantification (LOQ), unless other evidence indicates a zero residue. Similar data are available from the web pages of some large food companies and supermarkets and other national authorities, as well as the EU (http://europa.eu.int/comm/food/plant/protection/pesticides/index_en.htm) and USA (e.g. http://www.ams.usda.gov/science/pdp/Download.htm, http://cipm.ncsu.edu/exportMRL). Some residues may be bound in the food and cannot be extracted by standard residue analysis. While this has been considered to be of no toxicological concern, because this residue was not bioavailable, more recent studies have examined the possibility of correcting maximum residue levels of highly bioavailable bound residues (Sandermann, 2004).

While agrochemical companies determine the MRL for major crops, there are problems in setting values for minor crops. In the USA, an inter-regional research project (IR-4) was set up to provide data for minor crop farmers (Baron *et al.*, 2003).

Before a pesticide can be registered, the MRL would be carefully compared with the ADI, the acute reference dose (ARfD) and the expected intake of the food. If the MRL value was too high, the pesticide would not be registered for use. The company that wished to market the pesticide may then perform further trials with a lower dose or extended PHI and, provided that it was still effective against the pest, it may be possible to register the pesticide with specific recommendations concerning the maximum dose permitted and when it may be applied. The MRLs in the UK are according to the Government regulations (Anon, 1999) as amended. If excess residues are found in a commodity, the producers can be fined and foreign imports banned.

An example of the decline in residue in a food crop is shown in Figure 7.5, where the MRL might be set at 1.0 mg/kg. Some large food companies will also carry out their own residue analyses to ensure that their suppliers follow the codes of practice that they set. Some supermarkets prohibit certain pesticides from being used on produce being marketed by them, or severely restrict their use. Many of these are the older, highly persistent pesticides, while others include organophosphate insecticides. Residue data obtained by a food company or supermarket are often displayed on their web pages. One crop that has been under surveillance, because a high proportion of samples tested contained residues, is pears. In 2002, 81% of UK samples and 66% of imported pears contained pesticide residues, but levels of chlormequat (a gibberellin biosynthesis inhibitor thought to increase flowering and fruit yields) have dropped as growers have ceased to use it. Residues of fungicides, notably carbendazim, have also declined with changes in pesticide usage and storage practice. The increase in the amount of food imported into the UK from tropical countries has caused concern as there has been generally less regulation of pesticide use. One example of a problem is where high residues have been found on yams treated post-harvest with a fungicide.

MRLs for food commodities in international trade are set by the Codex Alimentarius Commission (Codex), established jointly by the FAO and WHO as an international inter-governmental food standard organisation (Van Eck, 2004). Generally permitted legal limits for residues in food are based on the 'as low as reasonably achievable' (ALARA) principle. MRLs within the EU have now been harmonised, and extended to crops not necessarily grown within the EU, and this is anticipated to have an effect on the export crops of

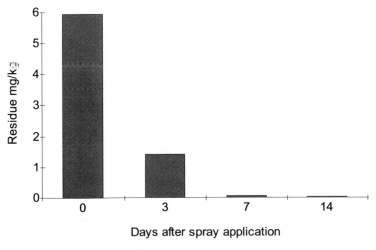

Fig. 7.5   Example of decline in residues following a pesticide application.

ACP (Africa, Caribbean and Pacific) regions. Where there are no appropriate data from GAP to derive an MRL, the LOD (Limit of Detection) is used. This has resulted in some pesticides being withdrawn as manufacturers have decided that the cost of generating the necessary field and safety data is not justified by the market for their product. To assist these countries, there is a Pesticide Initiative Programme (PIP) that provides protocols and advice to growers and exporters of fresh produce to assist them in complying with changing standards and regulations.

When the MRL data are published, newspapers often give headline prominence to the number of samples that exceed the MRL, even when it may be a small fraction of those analysed. It is important to realise that even when a residue in a sample exceeds the MRL, the amount of pesticide ingested will depend on the quantity of the residue-containing food that is eaten, and this value is normally far below the ADI. In most situations it is also true that a person would not eat the same quantity of the same food daily for their entire life. To obtain some idea of the worst possible scenarios of residue intake, three estimates are used in risk assessments (Renwick, 2002). These are: the TMDI (theoretical maximum daily intake); the NEDI (national estimated daily intake); and the NESTI (national estimate of short-term intake). Guidelines for predicting the dietary intake of pesticide residues have been published by WHO (1997), and provide a method of reaching reasonable assurance that the intakes of pesticide residues for different populations do not exceed safety limits. The guidelines also describe procedures that can be used by national authorities to predict the dietary intake of pesticide residues and decide the acceptability of MRLs from a public health point of view. Low *et al.* (2004) examined the published residue data and ranked results in various ways, concluding that there was no common trend because there is no single pesticide of particular concern from a consumer exposure viewpoint.

The TMDI is not easy to determine because it is based on a high long-term consumption of a food and the MRL, corrected for loss of residue during transport, storage and processing or cooking prior to consumption. Where a food is processed or cooked, the intake must consider only the residue in that part of the food that is eaten. Where a residue is mainly on the outer surface of a food, washing or peeling of the food could reduce the residue intake. Washing with water, for example, will remove some surface deposits, but a residue (particularly of systemic pesticides) can remain in the bulk of the food item. The amount removed from the surface will depend on the physicochemical properties of the pesticide, but gentle rubbing of the surface by hand, while washing, will assist the removal of deposits. Peeling or trimming vegetables and fruit can significantly remove surface residues. A change in residue in a processed food compared to the raw agricultural commodity (RAC) is referred to as a transfer factor (Table 7.2). As an example, if olives contain a residue of 0.5 mg/kg and the extracted olive oil has 0.2

Table 7.2 Some examples of transfer factors (from Timme and Walz-Tylla, 2004)

Crop	Pesticide	Process	Transfer factor
Apple	captan	ozone wash	0
		juice	0.1–0.3
		dry pomace	2–4
	pirimicarb	washed	0.7
Banana	tebuconazole	peel	1–2
		pulp	0.8–1
Buckwheat	malathion	noodles	0.4
Carrot	chlorfenvinphos	peeling/trimming	0.2
Orange	profenophos	peel	3
		pulp	<0.1
Tomato	pirimicarb	washed	0.6
	buprofezin	juice	0.1
		dry pomace	34
Wheat	bifenthrin	bran	3–4
		flour	0.3
		bread	0.1
		wholemeal flour	0.8–0.9
		wholemeal bread	0.2–0.3

mg/kg, then the transfer factor is 0.2/0.5 = 0.4. Transfer factors <1 indicate reduced residues, whereas a value >1 occurs if the residue is concentrated by the processing of the RAC. In determining transfer factors, samples containing residues similar to the MRL are needed to obtain measurable residues. However, the registration of a product will be made only if the residue level is sufficiently low, that there is no need to wash or peel the food item.

Where the same pesticide may be used on different crops, the TMDI has to refer to the mean intake of the different foods (Table 7.3). The TMDI is very much a theoretical value, but where it is less than the ADI, the possibility of the ADI being exceeded is extremely unlikely.

Changes in diet will influence the TMDI calculated for different regions of the world (Table 7.4). In an example, given by WHO (1997), the TMDI for the herbicide 2,4-D varied from 7 to 50% of the ADI.

Table 7.3 Example of TMDI calculation for an insecticide tebufenozide (from WHO (1997))

Commodity	MRL (mg/kg)	Diet (g/day)	TMDI
Grapes	0.5	18.02	0.0090
Husked rice	0.1	12.00	0.0012
Pome fruits	1	45.00	0.0450
Potato	0.5	240.00	0.12
Walnuts	0.05	1.00	0.0001
Total			0.18

Percentage of ADI = 16%.

Table 7.4   Example of TMDI from different regions (WHO, 1997)

Region	Diet (g/day)*	TMDI	TMDI (as % of ADI)
European	178.00	0.2744	46%
Latin American	116.75	0.1974	33%
Far Eastern	114.83	0.0961	16%
Middle Eastern	327.25	0.1636	50%
African	28.33	0.0447	7%

*Based on barley, black cherries, citrus fruits, eggs, maize, meat, milk products, milks, oats, potato, raspberries, rice, rye, sorghum and wheat. MRL at LOD.

A better estimate of the long-term intake of pesticide residues is derived from the NEDI, which is the sum for all food commodities of the intake of the food commodity times the relevant residue level of the commodity and corrected for any change in residue level caused by processing or cooking. This residue level is not the MRL, but a median level is determined in supervised trials (STMR), when applying the maximum permitted dose under GAP. Where the median residue is below the LOD, the latter term is used to calculate the NEDI.

Where a crop is seasonal, short-term intakes may be greater than the average. The risk is assessed using NESTI, derived from single-day consumption data, but this is complicated by possible variations between samples of the commodity. A person may consume a higher residue on a single occasion or day, because a certain food has a higher residue than average, or the person eats more food with residues in one day. Eating a large portion of food with a high residue would be the worst case. In practice, a consumer is unlikely to eat more than one commodity, such as a carrot, which happens to have a high residue on the same day. If the commodity is well mixed during processing, NESTI is calculated from the amount of the commodity eaten times the residue corrected for processing (e.g. peeling) and then divided by the body weight. This value would then be compared with the appropriate ARfD (Table 7.5).

The amount and type of food consumed by individuals varies, so estimates are made not only for adults but also for infants, toddlers (aged 1.5–4.5 years),

Table 7.5   Residue level (mg/kg) in the edible portion of a single unit of food commodities required to be eaten by a 60-kg person to ingest the ARfD

Commodity	Unit weight of edible portion	Acute reference dose		
		0.0008	0.003	0.1
Apple	127	0.4	1.4	47
Carrot	89	0.5	2.0	67
Peach	99	0.5	1.8	14
Potato	160	0.3	1.1	38
Tomato	123	0.4	1.5	49

children and adults. Certain foods eaten by adults have been excluded from the example in Table 7.6, which shows that the lower weight of younger persons is reflected by a higher NEDI.

As children have a higher rate of metabolism, have less-mature immune systems, eat different foods and consume more food per body mass than adults, their exposure to pesticides has caused concern. In the UK, an extra safety factor was proposed in relation to infant foods (Schilter *et al.*, 1996) to allow for the extra sensitivity of infants to toxicants, especially neurotoxins. In a study in the USA (Fenske *et al.*, 2002), the diets of two small groups of children of pre-school age were sampled for 15 targeted organophosphate insecticides. Among the 88 samples of food, which were divided into fruit and vegetables, beverages, processed foods and dairy products, 16 samples had a detectable residue of at least one organophosphate, with two of these samples having residues of two insecticides. Only in one sample was the acute population-adjusted reference dose (aPAD) for chlorpyrifos (1.7 µg/kg/day) exceeded, whereas in all other cases the exposure was up to 0.24 µg/kg/day. Other routes of exposure were not assessed in this study, so the children could get a higher dose from contaminated surfaces in their house or garden.

Some of the residues found in crops may be due to treatment either shortly before harvest, or during storage. Some crops are sprayed close to harvest with fungicides to reduce potential losses due to disease in marketing and storage, while insecticides may be applied in stores.

Problems have arisen due to variation within samples, although in making assessments it is usual to assume that the total pesticide residue measure in a bulk sample is derived from one unit of the bulked sample. Thus, if a bulked sample of twenty carrots contained *x* mg/kg, it might all be in one carrot. When samples of fruit were examined, there was no correlation between the residue concentration or surface residue and the mass of apples (Ambrus, 2000). The view was that the residue distribution was most likely to be influenced by the size, shape and density of the plants and mode of application. Thus, the variability in the initial spray deposit was a key factor influencing the ultimate residue in the harvested fruit. In contrast, following the discovery that residues in carrots could vary by up to 25-fold in a com-

Table 7.6 Changes in NEDI between adults and children

	Adult	Child	Toddler	Infant
Body weight (kg)	70.1	43.3	14.5	7.5
Mean NEDI* (mg/kg bw/day)	0.000,047	0.000,057	0.000,091	0.000,114
Total NEDI**	0.0006	0.0007	0.001	0.009

*These example values are the mean of several individual foods for one insecticide.
**Calculated NEDI based on amount eaten as shown by surveys of diet.

posite sample (Harris, 2000), experiments with carrots could not identify any single factor that was the cause of high residues in individual roots (Carter *et al.*, 2000). The variations in daily intake of food that occur are not a normal part of consumer risk assessment, which is a limitation when there is an acute toxicity risk from a pesticide. However, probability distributions of residue in food consumed can be calculated using probabilistic modelling, with account being taken of the variability of detectable residues to give a realistic estimate of risks from short-term exposure (Hamey and Harris, 1999). Some of the residue problems that have occurred have been due to excessive doses being applied, poor calibration of equipment, too many sprays being applied, or overdosing due to overlapping swaths. The adoption of integrated pest management and using reduced dosages when possible also cuts down the risk of a pesticide residue in the harvested crop (Fig. 7.6). Non-compliance of PHIs and spray drift from adjacent crops have also been implicated. These problems are potentially more serious in developing countries that lack the training in correct application of pesticides (Matthews *et al.*, 2003). Efforts are being made to help developing countries, especially the African, Caribbean and Asian countries (ACP) through the PIP to meet the new standards for importing fresh produce into Europe. Retailers are using Assured Produce schemes that meet Euregap and similar standards.

Many of the residue problems of earlier decades have diminished as the persistent chemicals (e.g. organochlorine insecticides) have been banned and replaced by less-persistent pesticides. In endeavouring to produce food at

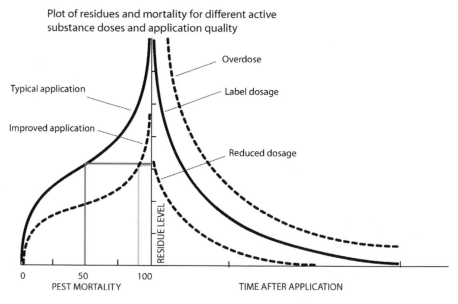

Fig. 7.6 Reduced dosage in field and subsequent decay of deposit to result in lower residue levels in harvested produce compared with label recommendation and overdosing (IPARC).

low cost and to avoid losses after harvest, some crops are treated close to harvest, and this is when produce is most likely to contain residues. There is therefore a conflict between the desire for chemical-free food and low cost (Foster *et al.*, 2003)

Risk assessments of pesticides have been made in relation to individual chemicals, but a crop may be treated at different times with a range of pesticides. Where farmers do use different chemicals – for example, an insecticide may applied with a fungicide at the same time to avoid spraying on two occasions, or different herbicides are used in a mixture to treat a range of weed species – the pesticides have different modes of action and operate independently. As a harvested product may contain the residue of more than one pesticide, 'The Committee on Toxicity' in the UK recently reviewed (Anon, 2002) the risks associated with mixtures of pesticides. It was concluded that there is evidence for limited exposure of humans to multiple residues and that such exposure occurs at low levels. An example of multiple residue is shown in Table 7.7, in which three of the chemicals – two insecticides and one acaricide – exceeded their MRLs.

The main concern of the public was the possibility of adverse reactions due to the 'cocktail effect', but there is no evidence of the occurrence of such combined effects in humans. Where a few well-designed experiments have shown synergistic or antagonistic interactions or additive effects, they have occurred at high concentrations or exposure levels, which are probably unrepresentative of real-life exposures. In one study, groups of rats fed a diet containing different daily doses of chlorpyrifos also received daily doses of four other pesticides – alphacypermethrin, bromopropylate, carbendazim and mancozeb (Jacobsen *et al.*, 2004). Co-administration of these pesticides did not enhance inhibition of acetylcholinesterase activity in plasma or the brain. Some effects were observed where combinations had been administered (e.g. increased liver and thyroid gland weights),

Table 7.7 Example of residue of several pesticides found in one sample of Velcore beans, imported from Kenya (data from Pesticide Residues Committee report on Sample 3238/2004, published March 2005)

Pesticide	Type	Residue found (mg/kg)	MRL (mg/kg)
Cypermethrin	I	0.2	0.5
Dicofol	A	0.6*	0.02
Dimethoate	I	0.2*	0.02
Dithiocarbamate	F	0.2	1
Omethoate	I	0.1*	0.02
Profenofos	I	0.05	0.05
Propargite	A	0.1	CAC = 20
Tetradifon	A	0.1	No MRL

I, insecticide; A, acaricide; F, fungicide.
*Exceeded MRL.
CAC, Codex Alimentarius Commission value used when there is no UK MRL.

but further studies would be needed to ascertain which of the pesticides caused these changes.

Total diet studies have been conducted mainly in the USA, Europe and Japan, but a few studies relate to tropical countries. Sawaya *et al.* (2000), when reporting pesticide levels in Kuwait, showed that in one cereal product fenitrothion did exceed the MRL sufficiently to warrant action. Most instances of pesticide poisoning due to eating food with high residues are rare, but when they do occur they have been due to misuse of a pesticide on a crop, for which its use is not registered. Aldicarb on watermelons in California was one example of misuse. The deliberate use of a rodenticide on a food, intended as a rat control bait, has also caused poisoning and mortality when the bait was eaten by humans.

There is considerable concern among some people that food contains any residues of pesticides. Should they be concerned? Even before any pesticides were developed, food contained a range of other substances which were not necessarily nutritious and, on occasion, might even be toxic. Plants have evolved an array of toxins as a defence system against attacks by insects and pathogens and to deter grazing animals. The hotness of chilli peppers is due to capsaicin, which is an anti-fungal agent and anti-feedant. A variety of potatoes, 'Lenape', planted by organic growers, had to be withdrawn due to their high content of solanine and chaconine, both of which are toxic to man (Fenwick *et al.*, 1990). There are monitoring programmes for some crops, such as potatoes to ensure that the safety level for natural toxins is not exceeded (Table 7.8). High-yielding potato varieties have been selected to be resistant to certain pests – for example, Maris Piper is resistant to some cyst nematodes but still requires pesticide protection from aphids, slugs and late blight (Foster *et al.*, 2003).

In the development of most of the major food plants, such as wheat, rice and maize, varieties have been selected with relatively few toxins so that they are palatable to us. The leaves of wild cabbage (*Brassica oleracea*), from which modern cabbage, broccoli and cauliflower have been bred, contain twice the amount of many glucosinolates as cultivated cabbage (Mithen *et al.*, 1987).

Thus, many foods that we do like contain substances that we refer to as 'xenobiotics' – that is, they are foreign to our bodies and are not nutritious. The stimulant caffeine in coffee is a good example of this, and in the USA

Table 7.8   Examples of glycoalkaloid content in certain potato cultivars (from Berry, 2004)

Cultivar	Glycoalkaloid content (mg/100 g dry weight)
King Edward	80–120
Pentland Hawk	90–130
Epicure	110–140

Note: potatoes with >200 mg/100 kg dry weight may not be marketed.

there is a legal limit of 6 mg caffeine per liquid ounce in beverages (the acute oral LD_{50} of caffeine is 150 mg/kg). However, as man has evolved, our bodies have co-evolved systems to break down small quantities of these xenobiotics so that they are harmless, or are excreted. A person taking a painkiller such as paracetamol will benefit from taking the prescribed dose, but the body cannot cope adequately from an overdose and too many tablets kill the patient (Lappin, 2002). Even in the sixteenth century, Paracelsus (1493–1541), a Swiss medical practitioner, noted that the correct dose differentiates a poison from a remedy. So, our body can cope with small amounts of pesticide in our diet and can metabolise them. The problems occur with an overdose, as in suicide attempts, or excessive exposure during the application of pesticides. As described in earlier chapters, before a pesticide is registered and allowed to be sold, it is extensively tested to ensure that when applied as recommended, any residue in the crop at harvesting will not be hazardous to eat. In contrast, some of the 'natural' foods would fail some of these tests (Ames *et al.*, 1990).

Some of the unusual chemicals in some foods are considered to be therapeutic. The flavinoids are one group of plant polyphenols, some of which are thought to play a role in maintaining health, although others may be toxic. Among these antioxidant phytochemicals are the procyanidins, found in several foods such as apples, almonds, barley, grapes, tea, maize, cinnamon, cocoa, peanuts, wine and strawberries. These procyanidins may modulate key biological pathways in mammals. A high-polyphenol diet has been shown in epidemiological studies to reduce the risk of coronary heart disease and stroke, by inhibiting the oxidation of low-density lipoproteins (LDLs). It is claimed that the risk of atherosclerosis developing is reduced by preventing LDL (regarded as bad cholesterol) from building up plaque in the arteries, while increasing the good cholesterol. Cocoa, chocolate, green tea, grapes, apples and red wine contain flavonoids, which are a specific sub-class of these compounds, and have also received attention as being beneficial to health. Culliney *et al.* (1993) provided a more detailed account of the question of natural toxicants in food.

According to the UK Food Standards Agency, fruit and vegetables should make up about one-third of the food eaten each day. It is also important to eat a variety, with 'five-a-day' as a good, achievable target. One portion is considered to be 80 g. The FSA considers that the risk to health from eliminating fruit and vegetables from the diet would far outweigh the risks posed by possible exposure to pesticide residues.

Farmers generally only use pesticides when it is economically justified to protect their crops and thus achieve a higher yield of marketable produce. Market forces with 'Assured Produce' schemes and similar programmes operated by reputable supermarkets and wholesalers ensure that if a farmer is to remain in business, then every effort will be made to ensure that any residue will be below the MRL. An extensive return to 'organic' produce without carefully regulated pesticides will inevitably raise the costs of commodities and increase the presence of lower quality produce with a short shelf-life.

The public is concerned about the presence of pesticide residues in foods. This chapter has shown that by sampling and by using very sophisticated analytical techniques, it is now possible to detect chemicals in extremely small quantities. The mere presence of these is not an indication of a risk to health unless they far exceed the MRLs, a level which confirms that the pesticide has been applied according to GAP. Regular checks ensure that the residues found in our foods are well below levels that would cause concern.

References

Ambrus, A. (2000) Within and between field variability of residue data and sampling implications. *Food Additives and Contaminants* **17**, 519–537.

Ames, B.N., Profet, M. and Gould, L.W. (1990) Nature's chemicals and synthetic chemicals: Comparative toxicology. *Proceedings of the National Academy of Science of the USA* **87**, 7782–7786.

Anon (1999) *The Pesticides (Maximum Residue Levels in Crops, Food and Feeding Stuffs) (England and Wales) Regulations 1999*, Statutory Instruments.

Anon (2002) *Risk Assessment of Mixtures of Pesticides and Similar Substances*. Committee on Toxicity, The Food Standards Agency, London.

Baron, J.J., Kukel, D.L., Holm, R.E., Hunter, C., Archambault, S. and Boddis, W. (2003) Co-operative facilitation of registrations of crop protection chemicals in fruits, vegetables and other speciality crops in the United States and Canada. *The BCPC International Congress – Crop Science and Technology 2003*, pp. 583–588.

Berry, C. (2004) Explaining the risks. In: Hamilton, D. and Crossley, S. (Eds.), *Pesticide Residues in Food and Drinking Water: Human exposure and risks*. Wiley, Chichester, pp. 339–351.

Carter, A.D., Fogg, P. and Beard, G.R. (2000) Investigations into the causes of residue variability on carrots in the UK. *Food Additives and Contaminants* **17**, 503–509.

Culliney, T.W., Pimentel, D. and Pimental, M.H. (1993) Pesticides and natural toxicants in foods. In: Pimental, D. and Lehman, H. (Eds.), *The Pesticide Question – Environment, Economics and Ethics*. Chapman & Hall, New York, pp. 1126–1150.

Fenske, R.A., Kedan, G., Lu, C., Fisker-Andersen, J.A. and Curl, C.L. (2002) Assessment of organophosphorus pesticide exposures in the diets of preschool children in Washington State. *Journal of Exposure Analysis and Environmental Epidemiology* **12**, 21–28.

Fenwick, G.R., Johnson, I.T. and Hedley, C.I. (1990) Toxicity of disease-resistant plant strains. *Trends in Food Science and Technology* **1**, 23–25.

Foster, G.N., Atkinson, D. and Burnett, F.J. (2003) Pesticide residues – better early than never? *The BCPC International Congress – Crop Science and Technology 2003*, pp. 711–718.

Hamey, P.Y. and Harris, C.A. (1999) The variation of pesticide residues in fruits and vegetables and the associated assessment of risk. *Regulatory Toxicology and Pharmacology* **30**, S34–S41.

Harris, C.A. (2000) How the variability issue was uncovered: History of the UK residue variability findings. *Food Additives and Contaminants* **17**, 401–495.

Hyder, K. and Travis, K.Z. (2003) Maximum residue levels: A critical investigation. *The BCPC International Congress – Crop Science and Technology 2003*, pp. 569–574.

Jacobsen, H., Ostergaard, G., Lam, H.R., Poulsen, M.E., Frandsen, H., Ladefoged, O. and Meyer, O. (2004) Repeated dose 28-day oral toxicity study in Wistar rats with a mixture of five pesticides often found as residues in food: Alphacypermethrin, bromopropylate, carbendazim, chlorpyrifos and mancozeb. *Food and Chemical Toxicology* **42**, 1269–1277.

Lappin, G. (2002) Chemical toxins and body defences. *Biologist* **49**, 33–37.

Low, F., Lin, H.-M., Gerrard, J.A., Cressey, P.J. and Shaw, I.C. (2004) Ranking the risk of pesticide dietary intake. *Pest Management Science* **60**, 842–848.

Matthews, G.A., Dobson, H.M., Wiles, T.L. and Warburton, H. (2003) *The Impact of Pesticide Application Equipment and its Use in Developing Countries, with Particular Reference to Residues in Food, Environmental Effects and Human Safety*. FAO.

Mithen, R.F., Lewis, B.G., Heany R.K. and Fenwick, G.R. (1987) *Phytochemistry* **26**, 1969–1973.

Renwick, A.G. (2002) Pesticide residue analysis and its relationship to hazard characterisation (ADI/ARfD) and intake estimations (NEDI/NESTI). *Pest Management Science* **58**, 1073–1082.

Sandermann, H. (2004) Bound and unextractable pesticide plant residues: chemical characterization and consumer exposure. *Pest Management Science* **60**, 613–623.

Sawaya, W.N., Al-Awadhi, F.A., Saeed, T., Al-Omair, A., Husain, A., Ahmad, N., Al-Omirah, H., Al-Zenki, S., Khalafawi, S., Al-Otaibi, J. and Al-Amiri, H. (2000) Dietary intake of organophosphate pesticides in Kuwait. *Food Chemistry* **69**, 331–338.

Schilter, B., Renwick, A.G. and Huggett, A.C. (1996) Limits for pesticide residues in infant foods: A safety-based proposal. *Regulatory Toxicology and Pharmacology* **24**, 126–140.

Timme, G. and Walz-Tylla, B. (2004) Effects of food preparation and processing on pesticide residues in commodities of plant origin. In: Hamilton, D. and Crossley, S. (Eds.), *Pesticide Residues in Food and Drinking Water: Human exposure and risks*. Wiley, Chichester, pp. 121–148.

Van Eck, W.H. (2004) International Standards: The international harmonization of pesticide residue standards for food and drinking water. In: Hamilton, D. and Crossley, S. (Eds.), *Pesticide Residues in Food and Drinking Water: Human exposure and risks*. Wiley, Chichester, pp. 295–338.

WHO (1997) *Guidelines for Predicting Dietary Intake of Pesticide Residues*. WHO/FSF/FOS/07.7.

8 The future of pesticides

The FAO has stated that more than 840 million people remain hungry around the world. Even more suffer from micronutrient deficiencies. Thus so far, global efforts have not been sufficient to meet the World Food Summit goal of reducing the number of hungry by half by 2015. To make progress, modern agricultural technologies need to be used in order to feed and clothe the increasing human population. Without such technologies, the area of land devoted to agriculture would need to be increased, and this would cause serious ecological damage.

Weed management

Already about half the production of pesticides is devoted to herbicides as their use has replaced mechanical weeding. Research has developed hoeing equipment that can be controlled more accurately and by the use of in-line vision and GPS systems, but the movement of the soil does not always suppress the weeds and can disturb roots of the crop and increase the danger of erosion and soil degradation. Herbicides often offer a less-expensive way of suppressing weeds. The development of herbicide-tolerant genetically modified (GM) crops allows a broad-spectrum herbicide to control weeds later, after the crop is established, but before competition with the crop causes yield loss. However, regular herbicide usage is increasing the incidence of weeds that are resistant to particular herbicides. As with other types of pesticides, there is a need for a range of products with different modes of action, so that different chemicals can be rotated to reduce selection of resistant weed populations.

As in conventional agriculture, herbicide weed management is also an important tool for weed management in no-till or minimum tillage systems. These tillage systems do not count on the weed management function of the plough and also can only make reduced use of mechanical weeding such as hoeing or cultivating. By avoiding ploughing, they play a crucial role in avoiding loss of topsoil when heavy rain removes large quantities of soil, as well as preserving the environment of many soil organisms such as earthworms. Two widely used herbicides for minimum and conservation tillage systems are paraquat and glyphosate. Whereas paraquat has a rapid contact action on foliage (Bromilow, 2003) and the spray reaching the soil is adsorbed, reducing the risk of movement from the treatment area, glyphosate is slow-acting. It is very mobile in water, but is absorbed in the soil, where it can be degraded by biological processes. In advanced no-till systems using permanent mulch covers of the soil, herbicides do not even reach the soil; this is in contrast to conventional farming, where a considerable part of the herbicides ends up on bare soil surfaces. As soils under no-till produce less run-off, less leaching and are higher in organic matter, glyphosate does normally not create an environmental problem (Schuette, 1998; Jansen, 1999; Ruiz *et al.*, 2001). As for any pesticide, herbicides must be rotated with other products and other, non-chemical methods of weed management, in order to avoid herbicide resistance or the accumulation of the products in the environment. This applies even in plantation crops and no-tillage systems, where alternative weed control methods would include cover crops, mulch cover, mechanical controls such as slashing or rolling (Neto, 1993). Chemical weed control is an important complement in no-tillage systems and has contributed to their increased popularity. Where soils and crops are suitable for minimum tillage systems, the use of these herbicides will increase as adoption of the technique spreads to other areas of the world.

In the tropics, it was often considered that there was sufficient labour available for hand weeding, and governments were reluctant to use foreign exchange to purchase herbicides. However, the trend will inevitably be towards herbicide use as more people migrate to towns or, with the spread of AIDS, are too ill to do hard work. Weeding crops in the tropics is crucial in the early stages of crop establishment, and small-scale farmers have to limit the area of cultivation in order to cope with weeds during this period.

Disease management

Much has been done, and will continue to be needed, in terms of breeding disease-resistant cultivars. A change to a resistant cultivar can be relatively easy with annual crops, but changes in perennial crops inevitably have to be over a longer period. Even with some level of resistance, many major crops suffer from infections of pathogens and so require protection with fungicides. The production of high-quality produce that can be effectively stored is one situation where use of a fungicide at some stage prior to or at harvesting is often needed. More is now known about conditions that favour some of the important pathogens, so that by careful monitoring of temperature, rainfall, humidity and leaf wetness, the timing of a fungicide application, if needed, can be more accurate. Unfortunately, resistance to many fungicides has already occurred, so resistance management strategies are essential.

Insect management

Integrated pest management

Integrated pest management (IPM) has attracted many definitions since it was originally conceived as a means of utilising different control techniques together as harmoniously as possible (Fig. 8.1). To many, the aim of IPM is to avoid pesticides and essentially to grow crops organically with biological and cultural control of pests. IPM has also been largely associated with endeavours to control either a specific pest or the pests on one crop, and often with an entomological bias. In reality, there is a need for cooperation within an agro-ecological area to adopt pest management covering all the crops and their major pests, in the widest context, within the whole area. Many key polyphagous pests attack many different crops and non-crop host plants within an area, yet historically there has been little attempt to combine efforts of different farms to work together against the pests. As an example, whiteflies, *Bemisia tabaci*, will infest a wide range of plants affecting horticultural crops such as tomatoes and other field crops such as cotton in a country, yet the efforts in the horticultural and agricultural industries have not been integrated.

IPM has to be understood in a wider context of the entire cropping system and environment, to avoid the use of pest management practices

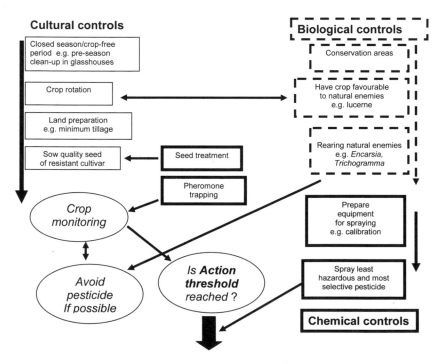

Fig. 8.1 Outline of different control tactics in an IPM programme.

that, although being non-chemical, have still a strong negative impact on the environment, such as burning of crop residues or ploughing.

Farmers find that outbreaks of pests can occur so intensively, and sometimes over extensive areas, that reliance on non-pesticide controls fails. Much depends on the crop, the cultivar, and where it is being grown, as climatic conditions can keep pest populations low in the areas with severe winters. In practice, pesticides will remain an important tool for farmers to maintain high yields. Their use, however, will become more selective both temporally and spatially, as farmers recognise the need to avoid blanket spraying of chemicals on a calendar schedule. Routine walking of the crop and scouting for pests has been advocated in many situations, so that a spray is only applied when strictly needed to avoid pest populations exceeding an economic threshold level. However, crop monitoring (Fig. 8.2a and b) must be simple and relatively quick to do; otherwise, its cost may not be justified by the farmer. Patch spraying according to maps of weeds has also provided a means of limiting the use of herbicides to parts of fields where specific weeds occur.

As pointed out by the agrochemical industry, in addition to making agriculture more efficient and productive on a limited area of land, research by industry is helping to conserve and enhance biodiversity. This is by promoting systems such as IPM or rather Integrated Crop Management (ICM) throughout the world. In one instance in Zimbabwe, it was referred to as IP^{2}M – Integrated Pest and Production Management – to emphasise the involvement of good agricultural practices for a high yield potential. In broadening the scope beyond the management of pests, ICM encourages protection of natural wildlife habitats within and around the farm. Globally, the aim is to establish a network of protected areas around the world as stipulated by the Convention on Biological Diversity. These areas include temporary (e.g. uncut field margins) as well as permanent conservation areas, within farming areas. In some cases, strip management or under sowing (Fig. 8.3) to conserve and encourage natural enemies, sometimes combined with releases of parasitoids or predators (see Fig. 8.2f) will affect pest population growth and may obviate the need for an insecticide spray. Mensah (1999) gives examples of habitat diversity with strips of lucerne alongside cotton, while Levie *et al.* (2005) give an example of aphid control. Many of these options have already been taken up by various schemes such as LEAF (Linking Environment and Farming) and some of the Farm Assurance Schemes which have evolved by closer partnership between farming and those marketing farm produce.

Traditional plant breeding

For centuries, farmers have retained seeds from good plants, which had survived pests and diseases, for sowing the following season. Then scientists

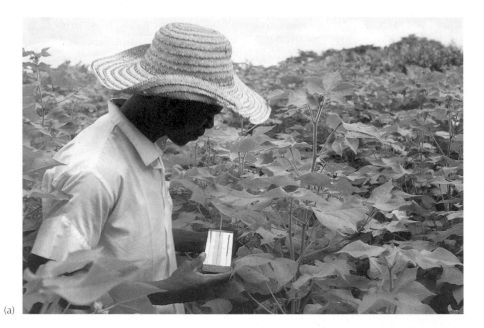

(a)

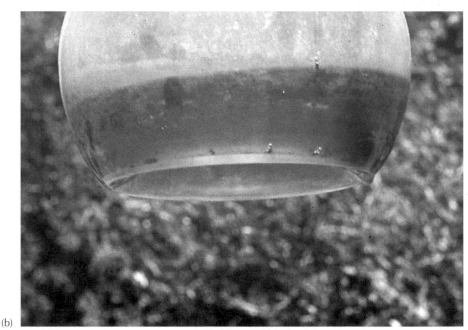

(b)

Fig. 8.2 Monitoring insect pest populations. (a) Scouting cotton; (b) trapping fruit flies. (*Continued.*)

made specific crosses between plants and selected those with the most useful traits to improve pest and disease resistance to achieve higher yields of better quality produce. It has been shown that, even with partial resistance to a pest or pathogen, crops may require less protection with pesticides. Changes in

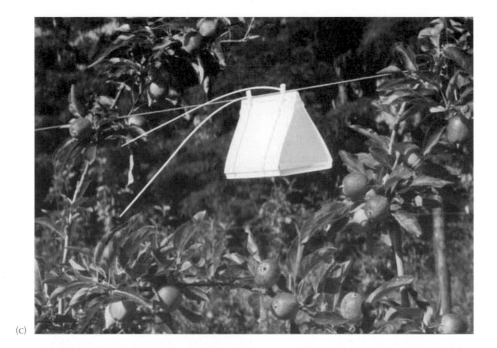

(c)

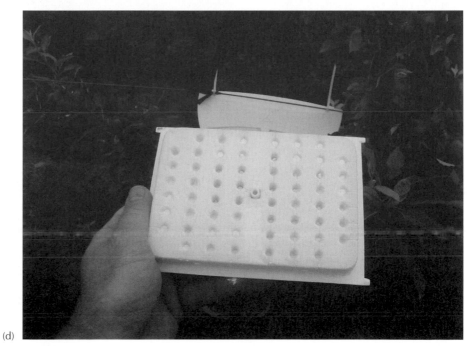

(d)

Fig. 8.2 (*Continued.*) (c, d) Pheromone traps (Exosect)l. (*Continued.*)

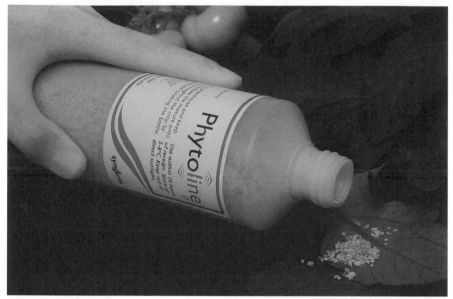

(e)

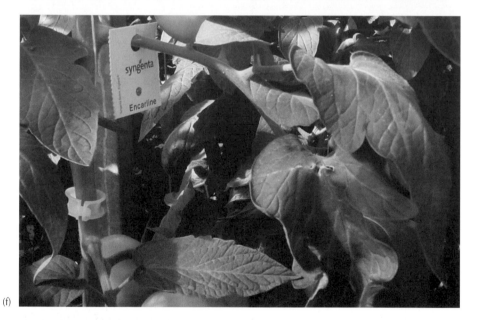

(f)

Fig. 8.2 (*Continued.*) (e); (f) releasing a biological control agent in a glasshouse (Syngenta).

the pathogen mean that a resistant variety may not continue to be effective, so plant breeders need to select new hybrids continually to keep ahead of the pathogen. The choice of crop variety continues to be an important component of IPM. Unfortunately, market forces often dictate the growing of varieties, which are more palatable to humans and produce a higher, more profit-

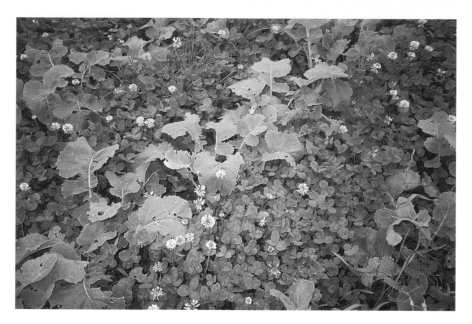

Fig. 8.3   Organic crop inter-sown with clover.

able yield, rather than putting the emphasis on pest resistance. Sometimes, despite great efforts to transfer a resistance gene into a food crop, the new cultivar fails as it is no longer as palatable or high yielding. Nevertheless, the selection of crop varieties by traditional methods is essential alongside the new technology of genetic engineering to ensure that in emphasising one particular trait such as herbicide tolerance, the variety is still suitable for the circumstances in different agro-ecological areas.

Present day pesticides

The agrochemical industry has changed significantly since the early days of pesticide development. While the older products no longer covered by patents have moved to generic companies, those investing in R&D have not only diversified into GM crops, but have also realised that the registration authorities are unlikely to accept the most toxic pesticides, nor those which are very persistent in the environment. In Europe, many of the older pesticides have been withdrawn as companies have declined to provide new data to meet the latest registration requirements. In some cases this has caused severe problems for some minor crops, for which no new pesticide has been registered, due to the small market for these crops. While broad-spectrum pesticides are needed with potential use of large areas of a major crop to cover the development costs, there has been recognition of the need for more selective products or more selective use of the broader spectrum chemicals.

Herbicides

Most new herbicides have been added to existing types, such as the sulfonylureas. More refined production has led to the *S*-isomer of metolachlor replacing the earlier product. In general, new herbicide products are often different combinations of herbicides in pre-mixed formulations to suit specific weed situations in different crops and countries. There has also been greater awareness of enhancing herbicide activity by recommending the addition of certain adjuvants, such as methylated vegetable seed oils, that improve the spread of the spray deposit on foliage and increase the amount taken up by the weeds.

Fungicides

The strobilurins, synthetic analogues of strobilurin A produced by *Strobilurus tenacellus*, have been the main new group of fungicides, although new versions of older groups continue to be developed. Prothioconazole is a new azole (Mauler-Machnik *et al.*, 2002). Ethaboxam is a new fungicide which is specific to controlling oomycetes such as grape downy mildew, and late blight on potato (Kim *et al.*, 2002).

Hewitt (1998) provides a detailed account of fungicides.

Insecticides

In place of many of the organochlorine, organophosphate and carbamate neurotoxic insecticides, new groups include the pyrethroids and nicotinoids. Other new groups are chitin synthesis inhibitors and other insect growth regulators as well as avermectin, milbemectin and certain other new pesticides, such as pyrazoles.

Pyrethroids

The pyrethroids are no longer new molecules, as they now play a key role in the pest control armoury. However, as they are a replacement of the organochlorine insecticides, reference to them is included here. During the 1930s and earlier, the natural pyrethrins extracted from the flowers of *Chrysanthemum cinerarifolium* were widely used to control insect pests especially in dark warehouses, where sunlight could not break it down rapidly. As mentioned earlier, scientists wanted to develop a photostable version of the pyrethrins, and this was eventually accomplished with the development of permethrin and subsequently cypermethrin and deltamethrin (Elliott *et al.*, 1973; Elliott *et al.*, 1978). Other pyrethroid insecticides have now been synthesised. These are reasonably persistent, and although the active molecule can be highly toxic to mammals, the amount of pyrethroid actually applied is extremely small – only a few grams per hectare compared with over 100 g or kg of older products. As with the earlier insecticides, once they become relatively inexpensive, they are used too often, with poor equipment in the tropics and by applying an overdose, selection of insects with resistance to them occurs rapidly. It is, therefore, important in any one agro-ecosystem to limit the number of applications so that only one generation of the pest is exposed to this group of insecticides. Even with use limited to a particular period – as practised in Australia on cotton – the insects might still increase their tolerance to the insecticide if other tactics in an IPM programme are not followed. Thus, the limitation of over-wintering populations is still important, for example where a closed season restricts the availability of host plants.

Neonicotinoids

The more recent development is this group of insecticides, which emulates the effect of nicotine derived from tobacco. These insecticides, such as imidacloprid, act on the acetylcholine system by blocking the postsynaptic nicotinergic acetylcholine receptors. The use of imidacloprid has expanded rapidly since 1990, both as a spray and seed treatment to utilise systemic activity against a range of pests including aphids and whiteflies. Similarly, thiamethoxam is recommended for control of these pests. Another new neonicotinoid is clothiaidin (Ohkawara *et al.*, 2002). The risk is that overuse of this group of insecticides will lead to widespread resistance.

Phenylpyrazole

Fipronil is an example of another new type of broad-spectrum insecticide used at very low dosages. It is also fairly persistent and must be used with caution. It is nevertheless an important tool in some pest control situations as it provides a different mode of action.

Insect growth regulators (IGRs)

In contrast to the neurotoxic poisons, these chemicals interfere with the growth of the immature stages of insects. At the larval stage of an insect, it moults and forms a new skin or cuticle. This process is controlled by hormones and requires the production of chitin that forms the skin of the next larval stage. IGRs can be categorised into three main groups: juvenile hormone analogues; anti-juvenile hormones; and chitin synthesis inhibitors. The latter group has been the most widely used and includes diflubenzuron. Larvae affected by this insecticide will start to moult into the next instar but fail to complete the process. The action is slow as no effect is discernible until the insect moults. Adults are not killed, but there is some evidence that oviposition is adversely affected if they contact a sufficient dose. These insecticides have an extremely low toxicity to mammals.

Juvenile hormone analogues, such as methoprene have been used to control mosquito larvae and have also been successful in controlling Pharaoh's ants in buildings, although the effect is not seen for some time after the application. Tebufenozide is an example of the anti-juvenile hormone type, which cause larvae to form precocious adults.

Spinosads

In 1982, a new species of Actinomycete was found in a soil sample from the Caribbean. From this *Saccharopolyspora spinosa* two fermentation products led to the development of new class of insecticide, the naturalyte class. Spinosad is the first product to be commercialised in this class. Its mammalian toxicity and environmental profile make it an excellent insecticide in IPM programmes. Spinosad is degraded by sunlight, but surface deposits become stabilised with activity at a range of pH values so it remains sufficiently effective on foliage to control a range of lepidopteran pests, yet it is safe to most beneficials. It has already been used extensively in conventional cotton crops to replace pyrethroids and to supplement control on Bt cotton.

Other insecticides

The quest for new compounds with different modes of action continues. Pyridalyl is a new insecticide with low mammalian toxicity, yet good activity against lepidopteran pests (Saito *et al.*, 2002). Another group, the spirocyclic phenyl-substituted tetronic acids, is showing promise with spiromesifen having activity against whiteflies and spider mites (Nauen *et al.*, 2002). Spirodiclofen has activity against mites and psyllids and scale insects, and offers an important tool in IPM fruit production (De Maeyer *et al.*, 2002). Another new systemic insecticide of low mammalian toxicity is flonicamid, reported to have a different mode of action and be effective as an alternative to organophosphates and neonicotinoids.

Bacillus thuringiensis *(Bt)*

While this is a bacterium, it is the toxin produced by certain genotypes that is very effective when ingested by certain groups of insects, as the alkaline conditions in the insect gut dissolves the protein crystal releasing the toxin. The spores are not toxic in humans as the pH of the gut is quite different. It is the gene that encodes for the toxin that has been incorporated into plants by genetic engineering (as discussed below). Apart from GM Bt crops, the *Bacillus* is also used as an insecticide, but it is only really effective if deposited on the foliage being ingested by the younger larval stages. There is no contact activity. It is an important insecticide in forestry and organic agriculture, and hence concern has been expressed by some people about its wider use in genetically engineered crops. *Bacillus thuringiensis* var. *israelensis* (Bti) has an important role in controlling the larval stages of mosquitoes (vector of the malaria parasite) and black flies that are vectors of onchocerciasis (River blindness).

Biopesticides

These are living organisms that are applied to crops in much the same way as chemical pesticides. The main groups of organisms used are fungi, viruses and entomopathogenic nematodes. Following the locust plague during the late 1980s, efforts were made to develop a biological control method. *Metarhizium anisopliae* var. *acridum* (Fig. 8.2e) had been isolated from a locust in Niger and was in the collection at Kew, but there was concern about whether the fungus would be effective if sprayed in arid desert conditions in Africa. As logistics dictate an ultra-low volume method of application against locust hoppers or swarms, the initial study with *Metarhizium* was to assess whether the spores could be formulated in oil and remain viable. Fortunately, the spores are lipophilic, so formulation in oil was possible and small-scale tests showed that locusts were killed by mycosis once infected with the spores, although it took a few days before death occurred. Infected locusts, however, would stop feeding and could also infect other locusts. Later studies showed that this mycoinsecticide was selective against grass-hoppers and locusts, so that in contrast to an organophosphate insecticide, the natural enemies – including birds – were unaffected, so control continued whereas where natural enemies had been decimated, immigrant locusts were able to survive.

Research has also shown that baculoviruses of insects can be effective, although there are problems of stability in sunlight and the need to deposit the virus so that it is ingested. Nuclear polyhedrosis viruses (NPVs) and granulosis viruses have been used in insect control. Purification of the insect viruses has been considered essential as crude extracts obtained from dead insects can contain other viruses that resemble pox-like viruses, but purification tends to make them more susceptible to ultraviolet radiation in sunlight. Thus, formulations of baculoviruses need to contain a sunscreen. Most success has been against forestry pests as delay in mortality and some damage has been acceptable, in contrast to horticultural crops. In Scotland, the pine beauty moth larvae were effectively controlled by baculovirus sprays, while in Canada the sawfly *Neodiprion sertifer* has been controlled by a NPV. Some research is examining the possibility of using baculoviruses as a means of delivering a toxin, such as the venom from arthropods to increase the effectiveness of the virus and increase the speed of action.

Larger living organisms used as control agents are the entomopathogenic nematodes (EPNs), such as *Steinernema feltiae*. As with Bt, it is a toxin that causes death, having been carried into the insect by the nematode. The infective juveniles (IJs) are applied, usually in large volumes of water to control soil pests, such as the vine weevil (*Orthorhinus klugi*). Care is needed when using conventional spray equipment to avoid damaging the nematodes by sheer forces in the pump or nozzle and high temperatures caused by recirculating the spray several times through the pump. Careful distribution is needed to avoid leaving sections untreated as the nematodes will not move through dry soil. Research has investigated the addition of certain polymers to permit spraying EPNs to foliar pests, by keeping sufficient moisture on the IJs for a longer period.

In the global market, after Bt, EPNs have so far been the most successful biopesticides as they are multicellular living organisms and thus do not have to be registered for sale as a control agent. A major hurdle for alternatives to chemical pesticides is the need to register pesticides. Many have advocated the use of botanicals, assuming that with a natural origin these are safer, but history has shown that botanical insecticides can also be highly toxic, as shown by nicotine and rotenone. The myco-pesticides may present quite different risks to users, such as a person's sensitivity to a protein, causing asthma or a skin reaction. Clearly, some registration system is required, although a softer approach is justified for some new techniques, such as the use of pheromones (see below) which are highly specific to certain organisms.

More selective applications

The continued supply of broad-spectrum insecticides has led to a need to consider more selective treatments where possible. Elsewhere, attention has been drawn to the need to avoid downwind drift affecting watercourses and natural habitats by careful selection of spray nozzles and use of no-spray buffer zones. The use of monitoring systems can assist in limiting the number of treatments and timing those that are needed to have the greatest impact on a pest population. When a spray can be directed at the most susceptible stage – often the first or second larval instars – the dose that needs to be applied can often be lower than that given on the label.

Traditionally, most pesticide sprays are directed downwards on field crops. However, by angling nozzles forwards or backwards (sometimes in both directions with twin nozzles) it has been possible to improve deposition on the near-vertical stems of cereal crops and improve the effectiveness of fungicide treatments. Early crop establishment is important so that the crop can compete with weeds so seed treatment will continue to be an important technique for protecting young seedlings. Patch spraying was referred to earlier as it is particularly relevant to herbicide application where specific weeds can be mapped and treatments localised accordingly. On a smaller scale, spot treatments and the use of weed wipers also provides selective localised treatment of weeds.

In vector control, the treatment of bed-nets is a selective treatment in areas with malaria, as the anopheline mosquitoes are only exposed to deposits when attracted by the person sleeping under the net. Unfortunately, if other mosquitoes (e.g. *Aedes aegypti*) are active when people are not protected by the nets, the transmission of some diseases can still occur. Other uses of lures to attract insect pests to treated surfaces are discussed later.

In locust control, if locust hopper bands can be detected, it is possible to apply barriers of insecticide such that as the hoppers cross the treated vegetation or eat it, they accumulate a toxic dose. Before the 1980s dieldrin was used, but with the banning of this organochlorine it is now possible to use fipronil in non-crop areas. The aim is to treat a barrier of about 100 m wide separated by a distance of at least 600 m or more between barriers. The area untreated allows survival of non-target organisms that may be affected by the insecticide. With this technique, the overall dose is less than 1 g of insecticide per protected hectare. The application of a chitin synthesis inhibitor IGR, such as diflubenzuron, against hoppers is also recommended. IGRs are more selective, but are slower in action.

Pheromones

There are many chemicals, now usually referred to as semio-chemicals, which modify behaviour through communication between organisms. Among these are kairomones that signal between different species, for example by attracting a natural enemy such as a parasitoid to its prey. This may be the odour emitted by a pest-damaged plant or in some cases by a chemical, which is also a pheromone. The pheromones most used in pest control are sex attractants. Among the lepidoptera, the volatile odour released by a virgin moth, for example is a strong attractant that guides male moths, often very long distances, towards the virgin moth, so that mating can take place. Pheromones are highly species-specific and effective at incredibly small quantities. They may consist of several chemicals or isomers in specific ratios, with a similar mixture, but a different ratio being used by a closely related species. They break down rapidly, especially in sunlight, so do not leave any residues.

Several approaches have been tried to utilise pheromones in insect control. One approach is to use the pheromone in traps to monitor pest populations. Catches can show when an infestation is starting. Insect numbers in a trap do not directly relate to the size of a pest population as the proportion of insects trapped may decrease with a higher pest population. Results from monitoring with traps may indicate when a spray or some other control tactic is needed, or merely warn the farmer to monitor his crop by examining the plants.

A major technique to control pests is to release so much pheromone in the environment of a crop that males have great difficulty locating a female and mating – the mating disruption technique. This technique has been used to control pink bollworm on cotton in Egypt where 'twist-ties' (thin tubes containing the pheromone) were tied to about one in 100 plants. Pheromone was released over several weeks through the plastic wall of the tube. Another mass disruption technique was to formulate the pheromone in microcapsules, which are sprayed on a crop.

A more recent pheromone application technology is to use an electrostatically charged powder in small traps. A moth entering the trap becomes coated by the powder, which is then carried by the male moth when it flies from the trap. This Exosex Auto Confusion system allows a much lower dose of pheromone to be used, as only about 25 dispensers/traps are required per hectare. The Exosect system is now approved in the UK for codling moth (*Cydia pomonella*) (Fig. 8.2c and d) control in apple orchards, although it had already been used elsewhere in Europe. The pheromone disruption technique is highly selective and so must be used in conjunction with other control measures needed in a crop, but the number of insecticide sprays is reduced.

Mass disruption of mating may well integrate with the adoption of GM crop technology as the method may reduce mating of insects with resistance to the toxin in, for example, Bt transgenic crops and supplement the impact of mating with susceptible insects outside the crop area.

Another approach is to use the pheromone as an attractant to an insecticide deposit – the 'lure and kill' technique. One successful example is the use of grandlure, the pheromone of the boll weevil (*Anthonomus grandis*), which is attractive to both males and females. Placing the pheromone with an insecticide on 'weevil sticks' placed around cotton fields attracts weevils emerging after the winter resting stage (from diapause) (Brashear, 1997). Lure and kill has been successfully used in several government control programmes against boll weevil, such as USA, Nicaragua, Paraguay and other, mostly Latin American cotton-growing countries, and offers possibilities of minimising insecticide use (Daxl *et al.*, 1995; Plato and Plato, 1997; Villavaso *et al.*, 2002). Tsetse flies have been effectively controlled by placing a plastic vial of octanol on screens of material dipped in insecticide. The odour of octanol is a strong attractant to get the flies to sit on the treated surface. Where there are herds of cattle, the direct treatment of the animal's skin with a pyrethroid has also been effective by using the animal as the attractant.

Most of the alternatives to pesticides considered here have only been successful in a limited area against specific pests. While there is scope for research to extend their application to other pests and crops, the relatively low cost of pesticides makes it difficult to justify additional costs and management skills needed to fully implement newer techniques. Much depends on the availability of pesticides at an acceptable cost to farmers and society. The reduction in active ingredients within the EU has stimulated more consideration of alternative technologies, but for the foreseeable future pesticides will still remain a key weapon in pest management. The last section in this chapter deals with a specific new technology, the use of GM crops. While the public has been reluctant to accept the new technology, at least in Europe, the area of GM crops continues to increase in many areas of the world.

GM crops

One clear advantage of incorporating a gene into a plant in order to increase its resistance to insect pests is that there should be less spraying of insecticides or even no need to apply certain pesticides to the crop. In one sense, the use of a gene expressing a toxin within the plants such as the Bt gene is a novel application technique, while also being a form of varietal resistance. The early data were not entirely clear as expression of the Bt toxin allowed some targeted insect pests to survive, but as the knowledge in gene transfer has improved, so far the GM Bt crops have enabled farmers to reduce their use of insecticides against lepidopterous pests, notably the bollworms and especially *Helicoverpa* spp., although some sprays may be needed for 'sucking' pests such as aphids. Where fewer broad-spectrum insecticides are applied against lepidopterans (e.g. bollworms), there is greater survival of predators, so biological control has a better chance against the sucking pests.

This reduction in 'bollworm' sprays on cotton has already had an impact. In China, farmers were sometimes spraying on more than eighteen occasions per season, using small, poor-quality knapsack sprayers, and often using insecticides classified by WHO as the most toxic. Hossain *et al.* (2004) referred to the period 1992–1996 when there were on average 54,000 cases of poisoning of farmers or their workers each year, 490 cases being fatal. However, since the introduction of Bt cotton only 9% of those farmers growing it have reported poisoning, in contrast to 33% of farmers who grow non-Bt cotton. The view was that, rather than criticising the adoption of GM crops due to perceptions on some speculative harmful effects, policy-makers should note the positive benefits of reducing the known risks of poisoning when using highly toxic pesticides. However, it is important to emphasise that when a GM variety is introduced, it must not be more susceptible to other pests. Where some Bt cotton has been grown, yields were lower, as jassids and other pests not affected by Bt caused severe damage.

Already since 1996, over 75% of the cotton-growing area in the USA is now sown with GM varieties. Many other countries, including China and more recently India, have recognised the value of GM cotton and increased the area with these new varieties, although debate persists regarding the usefulness of some new varieties and their efficacy in relation to the overall pest complex. Increasingly, these new varieties have several different genes stacked in them. Competition between commercial companies with the new biotechnology is introducing genes expressing different innovative traits, such as herbicide resistance as well as protection from insect pests. The combination of two *Bacillus thuringiensis* (Bt) proteins – Cry1F and Cry1Ac – in cotton plants extends the control of lepidopteran cotton pests, thus providing improved season-long protection.

Similarly, the sowing of GM oil-seed rape (*Canola*) expressing resistance to certain herbicides, especially glyphosate, has increased to over 75% of the world-wide area. It has been claimed that this has reduced herbicide use by 40% as the new herbicide-resistant varieties require only one or two applications of the single broad-spectrum herbicide, whereas more traditional unmodified crops need several applications of herbicides, often applied as mixtures. Other studies have suggested that herbicide use is not greatly reduced, presumably because of the weeds present and their time of emergence within a crop. The application of herbicides to GM herbicide-resistant crops is after crop establishment, so in most cases they can be applied more accurately to specific weed-infested areas, thus providing savings for the farmer and net benefits to the environment.

Hopefully, scientists developing GM crops will increasingly be able to develop cultivars resistant to the viruses and other diseases that are less easily or not controlled by conventional treatments.

Resistance to the growing of GM crops has been particularly vocal in Europe. In the UK, a moratorium on commercial GM crops was invoked, while large-scale trials were carried out to assess the effect of GM crops on biodiversity. Large plots of GM herbicide-tolerant (GMHT) crops of maize, spring-sown oilseed rape and sugarbeet were grown on large plots alongside equivalent commercial crops, treated as recommended with herbicides. The GMHT crops were sprayed with glyphosate (beet) or glufosinate-ammonium (maize and oilseed rape), when weeds were present and likely to reduce yield. Detailed records of the plants/weeds were kept, and observations were made of insects, including butterflies, and other wildlife in both plots at each site and in field margins (Champion *et al.*, 2003; Squire *et al.*, 2003). In these three crops herbicides did not have any major impact on weed diversity, except briefly immediately after a treatment. Weed seed densities were lower in GMHT beet and rape crops, whereas despite more weeds in GMHT maize, the seed returns were low irrespective of treatment. These effects in GMHT crops compounded over several seasons would, it was considered, decrease populations of some arable weeds significantly in beet and rape fields, although the reverse may occur in maize (Heard *et al.*, 2003). The changes in weeds could have an impact on many invertebrates, small mammals and birds, the populations of which interact with availability of their food supplies. Weed seed-feeding carabid populations were smaller in GMHT beet and rape, but larger in GMHT maize, while collembola increased with GMHT crop management (Brooks *et al.*, 2003).

In the row crops, no attempt was made to modify the application of pesticides. Instead of a band treatment leaving some weeds in the middle of the inter-row to be controlled later by tillage, the whole area was sprayed with a broad-spectrum herbicide. Leaving a strip of weeds on the inter-row until a later date was not studied, although in a separate trial different dates of applying herbicide was investigated in GMHT sugarbeet. Leaving weeds too long in the intra-row did compete with the sugarbeet, and reduced yields. In Denmark the weed flora and arthropod fauna was denser and more diverse in GMHT fodder beets in early and mid-summer than conventional beets when glyphosate was applied at or after label recommendations (Strandberg *et al.*, 2005).

Perceptions and hopes for the future

The general public tends to be wary about pesticides as they are acknowledged to be poisons and are used in such small amounts that they are perceived to be dangerous. This viewpoint is exemplified by the reports of the Pesticide Action Network (Craig, 2004). At the same time, the public accepts the everyday danger of venturing out on crowded roads where accidents occur far too frequently. Furthermore, the fuel used in our vehicles would not be accepted as a pesticide. It contains chemicals that cause cancer in laboratory animals, causes fire when ignited, and produces toxic gases (with very small PM10 and smaller particles) that pollute the atmosphere. Such pollution is not confined to cities, but affects everywhere with extensive roads. Many injuries and deaths occur and there are major costs in exploring, refining and transporting the fuel worldwide. Nevertheless, transport is needed so man accepts the risks, associated with the use of petroleum products. The change to using lead-free fuels is one response to the concerns of our polluted air, especially in built-up areas.

As with the Green Revolution of the 1950s, which was encouraged then to speed up food supply production and overcome the problems of famine in many parts of the world, there is a continuing need today for multidisciplinary research and extension to develop suitable packages of crop variety, whether GM or not, with the combination of weed, disease and insect pest management tactics that provide farmers with a profitable crop. Sustainable agriculture will require the judicious use of pesticides, and this can only be accomplished if the users are properly trained and the public educated to accept healthy food, even if minute traces of a pesticide can be detected. Regulatory authorities in many countries have now excluded most

– if not all – of the highly toxic or highly persistent pesticides, and with the agrochemical industry withdrawing support for many of the older products, the number of pesticides now available has declined significantly in Europe. Efforts by the FAO and others to harmonise the data requirements should lead more countries to follow the same principles and limit the number of active ingredients that can be used.

The European Union's Sixth Environmental Action Plan has set out an environmental policy for 2001–2010, which includes the aim of reducing the impacts of pesticides on human health and the environment. Many countries currently have – or will develop – a National Pesticide Strategy. Some of these policies, especially in Northern Europe, have aimed at reducing the quantity of pesticides applied or area treated. A 50% reduction by weight is easily achieved if a new pesticide is applied that requires one-tenth or less of the dosage of an older product. The new, more active molecule could have a similar impact on the environment – hence the need at the registration stage to assess accurately those physical and chemical properties and its toxicity, which can influence the spread and impact of a given product once it has been applied to a crop.

An alternative idea has been to assess the frequency of applications on a crop, but this can be influenced by seasonal differences affecting the incidence and severity of pests. Farmers with knowledge of local conditions may try to apply a lower dosage, but sometimes, if their forecast is wrong, they may need to repeat a dose; this will increase the number of applications, though the total dose may still be less than the manufacturer has recommended. Frequency of application can be a guide in certain areas where only a few crops and pesticides are used. Ideally, farmers would prefer fewer spray applications, as soil compaction will be less if there are fewer passages with the sprayer across the field. In some places using a modular system, tracks for the sprayer are retained, thus cropping is confined to definite beds.

With a wide range of crops, different products and seasonal variations in pest incidence, there is no simple formula for assessing whether pesticide reduction policies are effective. Overall, the need is to refine biological markers to assess the variation in bird and other wild animal populations, bearing in mind that these too are affected by meteorological and other factors. However, much has been achieved with improvements in decision-making to meet targets set by the supermarkets and retailers under crop assurance schemes. Better-qualified operators of pesticide application equipment, routine inspections of sprayers and more education of growers on the choice of pesticide will enable good yields to be obtained at minimal cost. The integration of non-pesticide tactics needs to be encouraged, but in many cases they will have a secondary role minimising pesticide use but not eliminating their use entirely on every crop. When used judiciously and only when really needed, pesticides will continue to be important in IPM/ICM. Figures 8.4 and 8.5 illustrate the processes of policy and improving

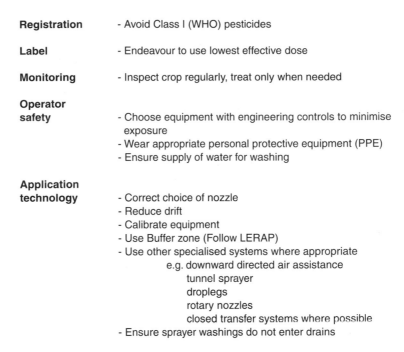

Registration   - Avoid Class I (WHO) pesticides

Label   - Endeavour to use lowest effective dose

Monitoring   - Inspect crop regularly, treat only when needed

**Operator
safety**   - Choose equipment with engineering controls to minimise
    exposure
- Wear appropriate personal protective equipment (PPE)
- Ensure supply of water for washing

**Application
technology**   - Correct choice of nozzle
- Reduce drift
- Calibrate equipment
- Use Buffer zone (Follow LERAP)
- Use other specialised systems where appropriate
    e.g. downward directed air assistance
        tunnel sprayer
        droplegs
        rotary nozzles
        closed transfer systems where possible
- Ensure sprayer washings do not enter drains

Fig. 8.4   Basic needs for using pesticides.

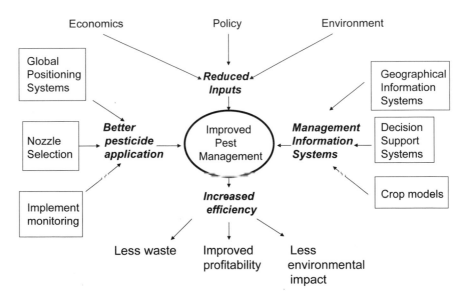

Fig. 8.5   Overview of improving integrated pest management (IPM) (adapted from a diagram by Franklin Hall).

information services linked with better application that can lead to more efficient use of pesticides within the context of IPM.

The dichotomy with IPM between the developing countries' poor resource farmers and developed countries is very wide. The latter are learning with government restrictions to endeavour to reduce chemical pesticide inputs, while there is a clear need to improve management of farms in many other areas of the world. International organisations have placed much emphasis on Farmer Field Schools (FFS) to empower farmers with more skills to improve their decision making. Agrochemical companies have organised stewardship programmes, but the sheer number of small-scale farmers means that these efforts often reach only a small proportion of farmers. Media attention to agriculture, consolidation of efforts and sustained inputs into better qualified extension service are all needed in order that better training reaches the farms.

In the past, many of the problems associated with pesticides have been due to the use of highly toxic or very persistent chemicals. Improved registration requirements have greatly reduced the availability of these pesticides. Harmonisation of data requirements and more education are needed to implement better application practices adopted globally and to reduce the adverse impacts of people's health and the environment. In summary, pesticides will remain a key tool in the pest management systems armoury. Indeed, GAP means more than Good Agricultural Practice, as *Good Application Practice* is essential to optimise dose transfer to where the pesticide is really needed.

References

Brashear, A.L. (1997) *1996 SEBWEP Baitstick Utilization Summary*. USDA-APHIS Report. SEBWEF, Montgomery, Alabama.

Bromilow, R.H. (2003) Paraquat and sustainable agriculture. *Pest Management Science.* **60**, 340–349.

Brooks, D.R., Bohan, D.A., Champion, G.T., Haughton, A.J., Hawes, C., Heard, M.S., Clark, S.J., Dewar, A.M., Firbank, L.G., Perry, J.N., Rothery, P., Scott, R.J., Woiwod, I.P., Birchall, C., Skellen, M.P., Walker, J.H., Baker, P., Bell, D., Browne, E.L., Dewar, A.J.G., Fairfax, C.M., Barner, B.H., Haylock, L.A., Horne, S.L., Hulmes, S.E., Mason, N.S., Norton, L.R., Nuttall, P., Randle, Z., Rossall, M.J., Sands, R.J.N., Singer, E.J. and Walker, M.J. (2003) Invertebrate responses to the management of genetically modified herbicide-tolerant and conventional spring crops. I. Soil-surface-active invertebrates. *Philosophical Transactions of the Royal Society of London* B **368**, 1847–1862.

Champion, G.T., May, M.J., Bennett, S., Brooks, D.R., Clark, S.J., Daniels, R.E., Firbank, L.G., Haughton, A.J., Hawes, C., Head, M.S., Perry, J.N., Randle, Z., Rossall, M.J., Rothery, P., Skellern, M.P., Scott, R.J., Squire, G.R. and Thomas, M.R. (2003) Crop management and agronomic context of the FarmScale evaluations of genetically modified herbicide-tolerant crops. *Philosophical Transactions of the Royal Society of London* B **368**, 1801–1818.

Craig, A. (2004) *People's Pesticide Exposures*. PAN, UK, London.

Daxl, R., Ruiz Centeno, B. and Bustillo Caceres, J. (1995) Performance of the Boll Weevil Attract and Control Tube (BWACT) in a 3-year area wide Nicaraguan Boll Weevil Control Program. *Proceedings. Beltwide Product Research Conference*, National Cotton Council, Memphis, TN, USA.

De Maeyer, I., Peeters, D., Wijsmuller, J.M., Cantoni, A., Brueck, E. and Heibges, S. (2002) Spirodiclofen: A broad-spectrum acaricide with insecticidal properties: Efficacy on *Psylla pyri* and scales *Lepidosaphes ulmi* and *Quadraspidiotus perniciosus*. *The BCPC Conference Pests and Diseases*, pp. 65–72.

Elliott, M., Farnham, A.W., Janes, N.F., Needham, P.H., Pulman, D.A. and Stevenson, J.H. (1973). A photostable pyrethroid. *Nature* **246**, 169–170.

Elliott, M., Janes, N.F. and Potter, C. (1978) The future of pyrethroids in insect control. *Annual Reviews of Entomology* **23**, 443–469.

Heard, M.S., Hawes, C., Champion, G.T., Clark, S.J., Firbank, L.G., Haughton, A.J., Parish, A.M., Perry, J.N., Rothery, P., Roy, D.B., Scott, R.J., Skellern, M.P., Squire, G.R. and Hill, M.O. (2003) Weeds in fields with contrasting conventional and genetically modified herbicide-tolerant crops. I Effects on abundance and diversity. *Philosophical Transactions of the Royal Society of London* B **368**, 1819–1832.

Hewitt, H.G. (1998) *Fungicides in Crop Protection*. CAB International, Wallingford.

Hossain, F., Pray, C.E., Lu, Y., Huang, J. and Fan, C. (2004) Genetically modified cotton and farmers' health. *International Journal of Occupational and Environmental Health* **10**, 296–303.

Jansen, A.E. (1999) *Impacto Ambiental del Uso de Herbicidas en Siembra Directa*. MAG/DIA/DEAG-GTZ, San Lorenzo, Paraguay.

Kim, D.S., Lee, Y.S., Chun, S.J., Choi, W.B., Lee, S.W., Kim, G.T., Kang, K.G., Joe, G.H. and Cho, J.H. (2002) Ethaboxam: A new oomycetes fungicide. *The BCPC Conference Pests and Diseases*, pp. 377–382.

Levie, A., Legrand, M.-A., Dogot, P., Pels, C., Baret, P.V. and Hance, T. (2005) Mass releases of *Aphidius rhopalosiphi* (Hymenoptera: Aphidiinae), and strip management to control wheat aphids. *Agriculture, Ecosystems and Environment* **105**, 17–21.

Mauler-Machnik, A., Rosslenbroich, H.-J., Dutzmann, S., Applegate, J. and Jautelat, M. (2002) JAU 6476 – a new dimension DMI fungicide. *The BCPC Conference Pests and Diseases*, pp. 389–394.

Mensah, R.K. (1999) Habitat diversity: Implications for the conservation and use of predatory insects of *Helicoverpa* spp. in cotton ecosystems in Australia. *International Journal of Pest Management* **45**, 91–100.

Nauen, R., Bretschneider, T., Bruck, E., Elbert, A., Reckmann, U., Wachendorff, U. and Tiemann, R. (2002) BSN 2060: A novel compound for whitefly and spider mite control. *The BCPC Conference Pests and Diseases*, pp. 39–44

Neto, F.S. (1993) Controle de plantas daninhas atraves de coberturas verdes consor ciadas com milho; *Pesq. agropec. bras. Brasilia* **28**, 1165–1171.

Ohkawara, Y., Akayama, A., Maysuda, K. and Andersch, W. (2002) Clothianidin: A novel broad-spectrum neonicotinoid insecticide. *The BCPC Conference Pests and Diseases*, pp. 51–58.

Plato, T.A. and Plato, J.C. (1997) Alternative uses of BWACT (Boll Weevil Attract and Control Tube) in Colombia, Brazil and Paraguay. *Proceedings, Beltwide Product Research Conference*, National Cotton Council, Memphis, TN, USA.

Ruiz, P., Novillo, C., Fernandez-Anero, J. and Campos, M. (2001) Soil arthropods in glyphosate-tolerant and isogenic maize lines under different soil/weed management practices, *Proceedings of the 1st World Congress on Conservation Agriculture*, Madrid, 1–5 October, 2001.

Saito, S., Isayama, S., Sakamoto, N., Umeda, K. and Kasamatsu, K. (2002) Pyridalyl: A novel insecticidal agent for controlling lepidopterous pests. *The BCPC Conference Pests and Diseases*, pp. 33–38.

Schuette, J. (1998) *Environmental Fate of Glyphosate*. Environmental Monitoring and Pest Management, Department of Pesticide Regulation, Sacramento, CA, USA.

Squire, G.R., Brooks, D.R., Bohan, D.A., Champion, G.T., Daniels, R.E., Haughton, A.J., Hawes, C., Heard, M.S., Hill, M.O., May, M.J., Osborne, J.L., Perry, J.N., Roy, D.B., Woiwod, I.P. and Firbank, L.G. (2003) On the rationale and interpretation of Farm Scale evaluations of genetically modified herbicide-tolerant crops. *Philosophical Transactions of the Royal Society of London* B **368**, 1779–1799.

Strandberg, B., Pedersen, M.B. and Elmegaard, N. (2005) Weed and arthropod populations in conventional and genetically modified herbicide tolerant fodder beet crops. *Agriculture, Ecosystems and Environment* **105**, 243–253.

Villavaso, E.J., Mulrooney, J.E. and McGovern, W.L. (2002) Boll weevil (Coleoptera: Curculionidae) bait sticks: Toxicity and malathion content. *Journal of Economic Entomology* **96**, 311–321.

Appendix 1
Some standard terms and abbreviations used in the approval of pesticides

Technical terms

Ach   acetylcholine
Ache   acetylcholinesterase
ADI   acceptable daily intake
ADME   adsorption, distribution, metabolism and excretion
ADP   adenosine diphosphate
ADR   European agreement concerning the international carriage of dangerous goods by road
AE   acid equivalent
ai   active ingredient
ANOVA   analysis of variance
AOEL   Acceptable Operator Exposure Level
approx   approximate
ARC   anticipated residue contribution
ARfD   acute reference dose
as   active substance
ASV   air saturation value
AUC   area under curve
BCF   bioconcentration factor
bfa   body fluid
BOD   biological oxygen demand
bp   boiling point
BSAF   biota-sediment accumulation factor
Bt   *Bacillus thuringiensis*
Bti   *Bacillus thuringiensis israelensis*
Btk   *Bacillus thuringiensis kurstaki*

Btt *Bacillus thuringiensis tenebrionis*
bw body weight
°C degree celsius (centigrade)
CA controlled atmosphere
CAD computer-aided design
CADDY computer-aided dossier and data supply (an electronic dossier interchange and archiving format)
cd candela
CDA controlled drop(let) application
ChE cholinesterase
CI confidence interval
CL confidence limits
cm centimetre
CNS central nervous system
COD chemical oxygen demand
CPK creatine phosphokinase
cv coefficient of variation
Cv ceiling value
CXL Codex Maximum Residue Limit (Codex MRL)
d day
DES diethylstilboestrol
DFR dislodgeable foliar residue
DMSO dimethylsulphoxide
DNA deoxyribonucleic acid
dna designated national authority
DO dissolved oxygen
DOC dissolved organic carbon
dpi days post-inoculation
DRES dietary risk evaluation system
DT disappearance time
DT$_{50}$ period required for 50% dissipation (define method of estimation)
DT$_{90}$ period required for 90% dissipation (define method of estimation)
dw dry weight
DWQG drinking water quality guidelines
ε decadic molar extinction coefficient
EC$_{50}$ effective concentration
ECD electron capture detector
ED$_{50}$ median effective dose
EDI estimated daily intake
ELISA enzyme-linked immunosorbent assay
EMDI estimated maximum daily intake
EPMA electron probe microanalysis
ERC environmentally relevant concentration
ERL extraneous residue limit

F field
F$_0$ parental generation
F$_1$ filial generation, first
F$_2$ filial generation, second
FIA fluorescence immunoassay
FID flame ionisation detector
FOB functional observation battery
fp freezing point
FPD flame photometric detector
FPLC fast protein liquid chromatography
g gram
G glasshouse
GAP Good Agricultural Practice
GC gas chromatography
GC-EC gas chromatography with electron capture detector
GC-FID gas chromatography with flame ionisation detector
GC-MS gas chromatography-mass spectrometry
GC-MSD gas chromatography with mass-selective detection
GEP good experimental practice
GFP good field practice
GGT gamma-glutamyl transferase
GI gastro-intestinal
GIT gastro-intestinal tract
GL guideline level
GLC gas–liquid chromatography
GLP Good Laboratory Practice
GM geometric mean
GMM genetically modified micro-organism
GMO genetically modified organism
GPC gel-permeation chromatography
GPPP good plant protection practice
GPS global positioning system
GS growth stage
GSH glutathione
GV granulosevirus
h hour(s)
H Henry's Law constant (calculated as a unitless value) (see also *K*)
ha hectare
Hb haemoglobin
HCG human chorionic gonadotrophin
Hct haematocrit
HDPE high-density polyethylene
HDT highest dose tested
HEED high-energy electron diffraction

HI   harvest interval
HID   helium ionisation detector
hl   hectolitre
HPAEC   high-performance anion-exchange chromatography
HPLC   high-performance liquid chromatography
HPLC-MS   high-pressure liquid chromatography – mass spectrometry
HPPLC   high-pressure planar liquid chromatography
HPTLC   high-performance thin-layer chromatography
HRGC   high-resolution gas chromatography
H_s Shannon-Weaver index
Ht   haematocrit
I   indoor
I_{50} inhibitory dose, 50%
IC_{50} median immobilisation concentration
ICM   integrated crop management
ID   ionisation detector
IEDI   international estimated daily intake
IGR   insect growth regulator
im   intramuscular
inh   inhalation
ip   intraperitoneal
IPM   integrated pest management
IR   infrared
ISBN   international standard book number
ISSN   international standard serial number
iv   intravenous
IVF   *in vitro* fertilisation
k   kilo
K Kelvin or Henry's Law constant (in atmospheres per cubic metre per mole) (see also H)
K_{ads} adsorption constant
K_{des} apparent desorption coefficient
K_{oc} organic carbon adsorption coefficient
K_{OH} hydroxyl radical rate constant
K_{om} organic matter adsorption coefficient
K_{OW} octanol–water partition coefficient
kg   kilogram
l   litre
LAN   local area network
LASER   light amplification by stimulated
LBC   loosely bound capacity
LC   liquid chromatography
LC-MS   liquid chromatography – mass spectrometry
LC_{50} lethal concentration, median

LCA   life cycle analysis
LC$_{Lo}$ lethal concentration low
LC-MS-MS   liquid chromatography with tandem mass spectrometry
LD$_{50}$ lethal dose, median
LD$_{Lo}$ lethal dose low
LDH   lactate dehydrogenase
LOAEC   Lowest Observable Adverse Effect Concentration
LOAEL   Lowest Observable Adverse Effect Level
LOD   limit of determination
LOEC   Lowest Observable Effect Concentration
LOEL   Lowest Observable Effect Level
LOQ   limit of quantification (determination)
LPLC   low-pressure liquid chromatography
LSC   liquid scintillation counter
LSD   least squared denominator multiple range test
LSS   liquid scintillation spectrometry
LT   lethal threshold
m   metre
M   molar
MATC   Maximum Acceptable Toxic Concentration
µm   micrometre (micron)
MC   moisture content
MCH   mean corpuscular haemoglobin
MCHC   mean corpuscular haemoglobin concentration
MCV   mean corpuscular volume
MDL   method detection limit
MEL   maximum exposure limit
MFO   mixed function oxidase
µg   microgram
mg   milligram
MHC   moisture holding capacity
min   minute(s)
ml   millilitre
MLT   median lethal time
MLD   minimum lethal dose
mm   millimetre
mM   millimolar
MMAD   mass median aerodynamic diameter
mol   mole
MOS   margin of safety
Mp   melting point
MRE   maximum residue expected
MRL   maximum residue level
mRNA   messenger ribonucleic acid

MS mass spectrometry

MSDS material safety data sheet

MTD maximum tolerated dose

MWHC maximum water holding capacity

N normal

NA defining isomeric configuration notice of approval

NAEL No Adverse Effect Level

nd not detected

NEDI national estimated daily intake

NEL No Effect Level

NERL No Effect Residue Level

NFU National Farmers Union

ng nanogram

nm nanometre

NMR nuclear magnetic resonance

no number

NOAEC No Observed Adverse Effect Concentration

NOAEL No Observed Adverse Effect Level

NOEC No Observed Effect Concentration

NOED No Observed Effect Dose

NOEL No Observed Effect Level

NOIS notice of intent to suspend

NPD nitrogen–phosphorus detector or detection

NPV nuclear polyhedrosis virus

NR not reported

NTE neurotoxic target esterase

OC organic carbon content

OCR optical character recognition

ODP ozone-depleting potential

ODS ozone-depleting substances

OES occupational exposure standard

OLA off-label approval

OM organic matter

OP organophosphate pesticide

Pa pascal

PAD pulsed amperometric detection

2-PAM 2-pralidoxime

pc paper chromatography

$\mathbf{P_0}/\mathbf{P_1}$ parental generation, first (author dependent)

PCN potato cyst nematode

PDE potential dermal exposure

$\mathbf{PEC_a}$ predicted environmental exposure in air

$\mathbf{PEC_{gw}}$ predicted environmental exposure in groundwater

$\mathbf{PEC_s}$ predicted environmental exposure in soil

PEC$_{sw}$ predicted environmental exposure in surface water
PELMO Pesticide Leaching Model
pK_a dissociation constant
pic phage inhibitory capacity
PIXE proton-induced X-ray emission
PNEC predicted no effect concentration
po by mouth
POEM Predictive Operator Exposure Model
POP persistent organic pollutants
ppb parts per billion
PPE personal protective equipment
ppm parts per million
ppp plant protection product
ppq parts per quadrillion (10^{-24})
ppt parts per trillion (10^{-12})
PRL practical residue limit
PSP phenolsulphophthalein
PT prothrombin time
PTDI provisional tolerable daily intake
PTT partial thromboplastin time
QSAR quantitative structure–activity relationship
r correlation coefficient
r^2 coefficient of determination
RBC red blood cell
REI restricted entry interval
Rf retardation factor
RfD reference dose
RH relative humidity
RL$_{50}$ median residual lifetime
RNA ribonucleic acid
RP reversed phase
RPE respiratory protective equipment
rpm rotations per minute
rRNA ribosomal ribonucleic acid
RRT relative retention time
RSD relative standard deviation
s second
SAC strong adsorption capacity
SAP serum alkaline phosphatase
SAR structure–activity relationship
SBLC shallow bed liquid chromatography
Sc subcutaneous
SC suspension concentrate
sce sister chromatid exchange

SD standard deviation
SE standard error
SEM standard error of the mean
SEP standard evaluation procedure
SF safety factor
SFC supercritical fluid chromatography
SFE supercritical fluid extraction
SIMS secondary ion mass spectroscopy
SOLA specific off-label approval
SOP standard operating procedures
sp species (only after a generic name)
SPE solid-phase extraction
SPF specific pathogen free
spp subspecies
sq square
SSD sulphur-specific detector
SSMS spark source mass spectrometry
STEL short-term exposure limit
STMR supervised trials median residue
t tonne (metric ton)
$t_{1/2}$ half-life (define method of estimation)
T_3 tri-iodothyronine
T_4 thyroxine
TADI temporary acceptable daily intake
TBC tightly bound capacity
TCD thermal conductivity detector
TC_{Lo} toxic concentration, low
TD_{Lo} toxic dose low
TDR time domain reflectrometry
TEP typical end-use product
TER toxicity exposure ratio
TER_I toxicity exposure ratio for initial exposure
TER_{ST} toxicity exposure ratio following repeated exposure
TER_{LT} toxicity exposure ratio following chronic exposure
tert tertiary (in a chemical name)
TGGE temperature gradient gel electrophoresis
TID thermionic detector, alkali flame detector
TIFF tag image file format
TLC thin-layer chromatography
Tlm median tolerance limit
TLV threshold limit value
TMDI theoretical maximum daily intake
TMRC theoretical maximum residue contribution
TMRL temporary maximum residue limit

TOC   total organic carbon
Tremcard   Transport emergency card
tRNA   transfer ribonucleic acid
TSH   thyroid-stimulating hormone (thyrotrophin)
TWA   time-weighted average
UDS   unscheduled DNA synthesis
UF   uncertainty factor (safety factor)
ULV   ultra-low volume
UV   ultraviolet
VLV   very low volume application
v/v   volume ratio (volume per volume)
WBC   white blood cell
WG   wettable granule
WP   wettable powder
wt   weight
w/v   weight per volume
w/w   weight per weight
XRFA   X-ray fluorescence analysis
yr   year
<   less than
≤   less than or equal to
>   greater than
≥   greater than or equal to

Various acronyms used for organisations, committees, publications, programmes and projects

ACP   Advisory Committee on Pesticides
ASTM   American Society for Testing and Materials
AU   Africa Union
BA   *Biological Abstracts* (Philadelphia)
BART   Beneficial Arthropod Registration Testing Group
BBA   Federal Biological Research Centre for Agriculture and Forestry (Germany)
CA   *Chemical Abstracts*
CABI   Centre for Agriculture and Biosciences International
CAC   Codex Alimentarius Commission
CAS   Chemical Abstracts Service
CCFAC   Codex Committee on Food Additives and Contaminants
CCGP   Codex Committee on General Principles
CCPR   Codex Committee on Pesticide Residues
CCRVDF   Codex Committee on Residues of Veterinary Drugs in Food
CE   Council of Europe

CIPAC Collaborative International Pesticides Analytical Council Limited

COPR Control of Pesticide Regulations 1986

COSHH Control of Substances Hazardous to Health

COREPER Comité des Representants Permanents

CPA Crop Protection Association

Crop Life International global federation representing the plant science industry; formerly GIFAP and GCPF

CSL Central Science Laboratory UK

DEFRA Department of Environment, Food and Rural Affairs UK

EA Environment Agency

EC European Commission

ECB European Chemical Bureau

ECCA European Crop Care Association

ECDIN Environmental Chemicals Data and Information Network of the European Communities

ECDIS European Environmental Chemicals Data and Information System

ECE Economic Commission for Europe

ECETOC European Chemical Industry Ecology and Toxicology Centre

ECLO Emergency Centre for Locust Operations

ECMWF European Centre for Medium Range Weather Forecasting

ECPA European Crop Protection Association

EDEXIM European Database on Export and Import of Dangerous Chemicals

EFSA European Food Safety Authority

EHC (number) Environmental Health Criteria (number)

EINECS European Inventory of Existing Commercial Chemical Substances

ELINCS European List of New Chemical Substances

EMIC Environmental Mutagens Information Centre

EPA Environmental Protection Agency

EPO European Patent Office

EPPO European and Mediterranean Plant Protection Organisation

ESCORT European Standard Characteristics of Beneficials Regulatory Testing

EU European Union

EUPHIDS European Pesticide Hazard Information and Decision Support System

EUROPOEM European Predictive Operator Exposure Model

FAO Food and Agriculture Organisation of the UN

FEPA Food and Environment Protection Act 1985

FOCUS Forum for the Co-ordination of Pesticide Fate Models and their Use

FRAC Fungicide Resistance Action Committee
GATT General Agreement on Tariffs and Trade
GAW Global Atmosphere Watch
GCOS Global Climate Observing System
GCPF Global Crop Protection Federation (formerly known as GIFAP)
GEDD Global Environmental Data Directory
GEMS Global Environmental Monitoring System
GIEWS Global Information and Early Warning System for Food and Agriculture
GIFAP Groupement International des Associations Nationales de Fabricants de Produits Agrochimiques *NOW* Crop Life
GRIN Germplasm Resources Information Network
HRAC Herbicide Resistance Action Committee
HSE Health and Safety Executive
IARC International Agency for Research on Cancer
IATS International Academy of Toxicological Science
IBT Industrial Bio-Test Laboratories
ICBB International Commission of Bee Botany
ICBP International Council for Bird Preservation
ICES International Council for the Exploration of the Seas
ICM Integrated Crop Management
ICPBR International Commission for Plant–Bee Relationships
ILO International Labour Organization
IMO International Maritime Organisation
IPARC International Pesticide Application Research Centre
IOBC International Organisation for Biological Control of Noxious Animals and Plants
IPCS International Programme on Chemical Safety
IPM Integrated Pest Management
IRAC Insecticide Resistance Action Committee
IRC International Rice Commission
ISCO International Soil Conservation Organization
ISO International Organization for Standardization
IUPAC International Union of Pure and Applied Chemistry
JECFA FAO/WHO Joint Expert Committee on Food Additives
JFCMP Joint FAO/WHO Food and Animal Feed Contamination Monitoring Programme
JMP Joint Meeting on Pesticides (WHO/FAO)
JMPR Joint Meeting on the FAO Panel of Experts on Pesticide Residues in Food and the Environment and the WHO Expert Group on Pesticide Residues (Joint Meeting on Pesticide Residues)
LERAP Local Environmental Risk Assessment for Pesticides
MS Member State (of the EU)
NATO North Atlantic Treaty Organisation

NAFTA   North American Free Trade Agreement
NCI   National Cancer Institute (USA)
NCTR   National Centre for Toxicological Research (USA)
NGO   non-governmental organisation
NTP   National Toxicology Programme (USA)
OECD   Organisation for Economic Co-operation and Development
OLIS   On-line Information Service of OECD
PAN   Pesticide Action Network
PIAP   Pesticides Incidents Approval Panel
PPPR   Plant Protection Products Regulations
PRC   Pesticides Residues Committee
PSD   Pesticide Safety Directorate
PUS   Pesticides Usage Survey
RCEP   Royal Commission on Environmental Pollution
RNN   Re-registration Notification Network
RTECS   Registry of Toxic Effects of Chemical Substances (USA)
SCI   Society of Chemical Industry
SCPH   Standing Committee on Plant Health
SCTEE   Scientific Committee for Toxicity, Ecotoxicity and the Environment
SETAC   Society of Environmental Toxicology and Chemistry
SI   Système International d'Unités
SITC   Standard International Trade Classification
TOXLINE   Toxicology Information On-line
UK   United Kingdom
UN   United Nations
UNEP   United Nations Environment Programme
VI   Voluntary Initiative UK
WCDP   World Climate Data Programme
WCP   World Climate Programme
WCRP   World Climate Research Programme
WFP   World Food Programme
WHO   World Health Organization
WiGRAMP   Working Group on Risk Assessment for Mixtures and Pesticides
WIIS   Wildlife Incident and Investigation Scheme
WTO   World Trade Organization
WWF   World Wildlife Fund

Appendix 2
Checklist of important actions for pesticide users

Drift reduction

- Choose the nozzle type carefully – Coarse spray quality? (*Check suitability of nozzle for applying pesticide to the crop/weed.*)
- Air-induction nozzle?
- Consider using an air-induction nozzle.
- Change to a coarser spray for the last downwind swath.
- Reduce the operating pressure.
- Use downwardly directed air assistance in arable crops.
- Check that the spray boom is not too high.
- Avoid too fast a forward speed.

Downwind protection

- Check wind speed: avoid too high a wind or very turbulent wind conditions, but also avoid very still conditions.
- Use the lowest effective dosage.
- Buffer zones.
  - near water   LERAP or similar risk assessment should be carried out.
  - residences/schools.
- Use hedge/windbreak: ensure they have appropriate porosity and protect these with a buffer zone.
- Use another tall crop to act as a filter.

Protect water (in addition to above)

- Do not prepare spray on a hard surface.
- Collect any spillage.
- Only mix the right amount for a spray treatment.

- Wash the sprayer tank in the field and use a diluted spray on the last swath.
- Wash the outside of sprayer by the bio bed.
- Use a bio bed to dispose of any diluted pesticide.

Protecting the operator

- Always wear overalls. If not available, wear long trousers and a long-sleeved shirt (*keep this set of clothes separate from normal clothing*).
- Choose the least toxic product which is effective against the pest/pathogen or weed.
- Wear gloves when preparing the spray and when there is potential exposure of the hands.
- Wear a hat.
- Wear a face shield when preparing a spray.
- Wear an apron to protect clothing during preparation of spray.
- Wear a respirator if applying a fog in an enclosed space (*always check the validity of the respirator filter*).
- Use ear protectors if the engine/fan noise is above 75 decibels.
- Have water available for washing hands.
- Have drinking water also available (*keep it well protected from the pesticide, and only drink after washing the hands and face*).
- Use a closed-transfer system if available.
- Launder any clothing exposed to spray separately from other clothing; if disposable overalls have been worn, dispose of them through appropriate waste disposal services.

Appendix 3

A note on the publication of the Royal Commission on Environmental Pollution Report and reply by the Advisory Committee on Pesticides

After this book had been written, the Royal Commission on Environmental Pollution (RCEP) Report, *Crop Spraying and the Health of Residents and Bystanders*, referred to in parts of Chapters 1, 2 and 5, was published on 22 September, 2005. The Advisory Committee on Pesticides (ACP) responded with a Commentary on the report on 6th February, 2006.

In their response, the ACP agreed with parts of the RCEP report. In particular, the ACP strongly supported the proposal for surveys of biomarkers for exposure to pesticides and other environmental pollutants in representative samples of the general population of the UK. They suggested that the value of such surveys would be significantly enhanced if they also collected information about potential determinants of exposure, so that the relative importance of such factors could be assessed.

They also agreed that there was a need for better training of general practitioners in toxicology; improved access of patients to expertise in the clinical management of illnesses suspected of being caused by pesticides; more effective systems for the reporting and monitoring of acute ill-health related to pesticides; mandatory training for professional spray operators; and mandatory testing of spray equipment.

The proposals for notification of residents and other bystanders about pesticide applications were supported provided that the detailed arrangements are properly informed by preliminary pilot work and consultation with stakeholders.

However, in their response the ACP considered that the RCEP's recommendation for compulsory 5 metre buffer zones alongside residential property, schools and hospitals to provide added protection against possible health risks from spray drift was a disproportionate response to scientific uncertainty. As set out previously in their advice to Ministers, the ACP viewpoint is that buffer zones around residential properties could be justified on social grounds, as many people do not like pesticides being sprayed right up to the boundary of their property, and this in itself may impact on their well-being. However, a decision to impose restrictions on spraying on these grounds would need to balance the benefits to residents against the disadvantages to farmers.

In contrast to the RCEP, the ACP thought that it was unlikely that pesticide toxicity contributes importantly to chronic fatigue syndrome or multiple chemical sensitivity syndrome, and were not aware of any regulatory organisation that set exposure limit for pesticides, allowed for possible risks of these syndromes.

Both the RCEP report and ACP reply can be accessed in full on their web pages.

The Government's response to the RCEP report had not been published when this book was completed in February 2006.

Index

abdomen 100

Acceptable Daily Intake 32, 33, 125, 128, 168, 172, 174, 175

Acceptable Operator Exposure Level 33, 127

acetylcholinesterase 100, 179

ACP 29, 34, 119

action threshold 186

Acute Reference Dose 33, 172, 176

acute toxicity 31, 40, 151

ADI 32, 33, 125, 128, 168, 172, 174, 175

adipose tissue 124

adjuvant 54, 192

adult 177

Advisory Committee on Pesticides 29, 34, 119

aerial sprays 113, 118, 124, 148

aerosol can 46, 64

African diet 176

Agricultural Chemicals Approval Scheme 16

Agricultural Engineers Association 44, 58

Agricultural Handlers Exposure Database 79

agronomists 25, 34

AHED 79

air-assisted spray(er) 50, 51, 117, 168, 203

airborne (droplets, spray) 112, 136, 151

air concentration 114, 128

aircraft 16, 21, 52, 112

air monitoring data 38

ALARA 173

algae 40

alligators 42

amenity areas 16, 25, 49, 59, 63

anilinopyrimidines 8

annex 1, 4, 17

anti-cholinesterase 23, 94

AOEL 33, 89, 127, 128

aPAD 177

application of pesticides 46

application technology 46, 203

approval of pesticides 30, 43

apron 82, 83, 96

aquatic organisms 145

aquatic plants 40

ARfD 33, 172, 176

arm 100

aryloxyphenoxy propionates 6

Assured Produce 178, 181

atropine 94

automatic harvesting 127

Bacillus thuringiensis (Bt) 15, 71, 74, 146, 194, 195

baculoviruses 195

band treatment 57, 201

barlet yellow dwarf virus 72

BBA 16

BCPC 33, 54

bed nets 36, 46, 124

bees *see* Honey bee

'beetle banks' 155

benzimidazoles 8

Bhopal 19

biobed 101

Biocides Directive 29

biofactories 21

biological control 21, 186, 190

biomonitoring 92

biopesticide 5, 162, 195

bipyridyliums 6

bird(s) 41, 42, 151, 152, 153, 154, 158, 160, 162, 195, 201, 202

birth defect 38

blood samples 124, 125

boom width 50

boom height 137

body 85, 89, 96, 181
body weight 89, 177
boots 84
bracken 145, 148
bread 175
breast cancer 124
British Crop Production Council 33, 54
buffer (zone, strip) 25, 65, 110, 129, 133, 134,
        136, 138, 142, 147, 148, 196, 203
bumblebees 154
butterflies 154, 200
BYDV 72
bystander 25, 108, 114–119

caffeine 180, 181
calcium chloride 73, 74
calibration 80, 186, 203
California 124, 127, 144, 180
calendar schedule 187
capsaicin 180
CAPER 156
carbamates 4, 94, 95, 151
carboxamides 8
carcinogenicity 31
carpets 120
cascade impactor 113
case-control 38
cattle 198
Central Science Laboratory 170
certification 35
chaconine 180
checking nozzle 80
child 177
child proof 70
children 177
chitin synthesis 5, 193, 197
chloracne 22
chlormequat 72, 173
cholinesterase 95
chronic fatigue syndrome 25
chronic/'sub-acute' toxicity 31
Chrysanthemum cinerariaefolium 5, 192
chrysanthemums 79, 127
closed transfer system 37, 96, 97, 203
'cocktail effect' 32, 179
Code of Conduct 17
Codex Alimentarius Commission 17, 173, 179

Codex Committee on Pesticide Residues 17
cohort design 38
cohort studies 38
cold fogging 16, 66, 68, 125, 127
collection efficiency 112
Committee on Toxicity 179
Common Agricultural Policy 129, 155
conservation headland 153
conservation tillage 15
container(s) 35, 36, 70, 95, 125, 126
    multi-trip 97
Control of Pesticides Regulations 17, 30
Control of Substances Hazardous to Health 17
cooking 174
COPR 17, 30
COSHH 17
cotton pads 85
Council of the European Union 17
countries
    Argentina 100
    Australia 153, 156, 193
    Belgium 158
    Brazil 34, 44
    Canada 39, 109, 148, 195
    China 10, 22, 199
    Costa Rica 94
    Denmark 158, 201
    England 109
    France 44, 115, 118, 144, 158
    Germany 16, 110, 114, 115, 133, 138,
        139, 142, 143, 144
    Holland 79, 127, 135, 158
    India 1, 10, 19, 144
    Italy 22, 158
    Ireland 14
    Japan 10, 124, 154, 180
    Kenya 90, 100
    Kuwait 180
    Malaysia 94
    Mauritania 162
    Nicaragua 198
    Pakistan 20, 144
    Paraguay 198
    Poland 15
    Saudi Arabia 162
    Senegal 161
    South Africa 23, 153

Spain 93, 124
Sri Lanka 22, 94
Sudan 162
Sweden 158
Tanzania 95
United Kingdom 2, 9, 16, 23, 24, 25, 30,
      31, 43, 44, 70, 78, 96, 108, 114,
      115, 118, 124, 133, 142, 145, 150,
      155, 156, 158, 159, 170, 172, 173,
      177, 179, 198
U.S.A. 2, 14, 16, 23, 24, 39, 78, 88, 94,
      118, 120, 122, 125, 127, 144, 145,
      152, 155, 172, 177, 180, 198, 199
U.S.S.R. 21
Uzbekistan 21
Vietnam 22
Zimbabwe 34, 82, 146, 187
coveralls 35, 79, 82, 85, 96, 98, 115
'crack and crevice' 122, 123
crawling children 120
crop canopy 50
crop monitoring 186
Crop Protection Association 25
crop protection certificate 25
crop protection management plan 25
crop rotation 14, 186
crops (and foods) 46, 109
    apples 14, 51, 73, 74, 156, 172, 175, 176,
        177, 181, 198
    bananas 14, 172, 175
    barley 181
    beans 179
    broccoli 180
    buckwheat 175
    bush 51
    cabbage 180
    canola 200
    cauliflower 180
    carrot 172, 175, 176, 177
    celery 172
    cereals 9, 54, 147, 151, 152, 196
    cinnamon 181
    clover 191
    cocoa 181
    coffee 95, 180
    cotton 1, 9, 11, 21, 23, 59, 71, 74, 75, 100,
        153, 156, 186, 187, 193, 199

    field 111
    fruit 9, 14, 175, 177, 181
    grapes 172, 175, 181
    kale 154
    lettuce 75, 169, 172
    lucerne 186, 187
    maize 9, 12, 181, 200, 201
    mushroom 172
    mustard 154
    onion 172
    orange 172, 175
    orchard 111, 117, 138, 139, 140, 144
    peach 176
    peanuts 181
    pears 173
    peppers 180
    plantains 14
    potatoes 14, 124, 148, 172, 175, 176, 180
    olives 174
    rape 200
    rice 9,10, 62, 144, 145, 154, 175
    rubber 6
    soya 9
    strawberry 172, 181
    sugarbeet 148, 159, 200, 201
    tea 181
    tomatoes 15, 16, 21, 169, 172, 175, 176
    tree 51
    vegetables 9, 14, 120, 177, 181
    vines 51, 88
    walnuts 175
    wheat 9, 72, 117, 147, 152, 175
crop walking 71
crows 125
cultural controls 186
cyclodiene 151

daily intake 32, 174
dairy products 177
Daphnia 40, 144
data package 30, 43
Decision Support Systems 71, 138, 203
DEFRA 25, 29, 34
Department of Environment, Food and Rural
      Affairs 25, 29, 34
Department of Health 109
deposit 100, 177, 192, 196

dermal 78, 79, 94
dermatitis 23
dinitroanilines 7
diet 174, 175, 176, 179, 180, 181
dioxin 22
Directive 91/414/EEC 4, 17, 29, 34, 78, 115
disease management 185
dislodgeable deposit (residues) 118, 126
ditch 133, 134, 136
DIX 136
dogs 31
dose 32, 40, 43, 72, 181, 202
dose adjustment 142
dose transfer 47
dosimeter 120
drain flow 143
drains 142, 203
drift *see* spray drift
drift potential index 136
drift reduction technology 129
drinking water 30, 144, 155
droplets 50, 53, 66, 75, 84, 108, 110, 116, 133, 148, 168
drum design 90
dust application 62
dye 85, 86, 111, 112, 115, 117

ears 85
earthworms 15, 40, 158, 184
EC hazard index 33
ecological monitoring 145
economic threshold 187
eco-rating 156
ecological relative index 156
EcoRR 156, 158
EDSP 42
EDTA 112
efficacy 43
eggshell 152
egrets 154
electrostatically charged powder 198
EMA eco-score 158
emetic 23
EMPRES 162
Encarsia 186
endocrine disruption 7
endocrine disrupters 41, 42

endocrine disrupter screening programme 42
endo-drift 109, 110, 144, 151
engineering controls 91
entomopathogenic nematodes 5, 196
Environment Agency 145, 150
environmental aspects 133
environmental information sheet 25
environmental estrogens 41
Environmental Protection Agency 2, 29, 34
EPA 2, 29, 34, 42, 144, 155
Epicure 180
epidemiological study 38, 39, 42, 123, 181
EPPO 161
EPRIP 158
erosion 15, 184
ESCORT 2 41
estimated environmental concentration 39
EU 24, 30, 133, 144, 145, 154, 173, 199, 202
Euregap 178
European diet 176
European Food Safety Authority 30
European Predictive Operator Exposure Model 78, 79, 87
EUROPOEM 78, 79, 87
exo-drift 109, 110
exposure 25, 33, 34, 38, 39, 76, 78, 79, 88, 89, 90, 94, 95, 99, 115, 155
    measuring exposure 85
Exosect 198

face shield 82, 83, 96
fans 50
far eastern diet 176
Farm Assurance 187
farm summary 157
farm worker 123
FAO 10, 17, 23, 99, 159, 161, 173, 184, 202
Farmer Field School 10, 204
farmyard 143
Federal Institute of Biology for Agriculture and Forestry 16
feet (foot) 84, 85, 99
fire risk 66, 70
first aid 94, 95
fish 40, 145, 160, 161
flavinoids 181

flooding 70
Florida 125
flour 175
flowers 120, 126
fluoroalkyl methacrylate 79
fluorescent dye 87
fog 56, 66, 84, 91, 125
fogging equipment 85
foliage 50, 56, 75, 127, 150, 168, 185
food 32
Food and Environment Protection Act 16
food chain 4, 44, 162
Food Standards Agency 33, 181
forest 15, 59, 113
Forest Service Cramer-Barry-Grim (FSCBG)
        model 113
formulation 41, 79, 108, 109, 136, 168, 195
Friends of the Earth 42
frog 7
FSA 33, 181
Fullers earth 94
fumigate 114
fungicides 8, 9, 18, 79, 151, 154, 173, 185,
        192, 196
    azaconazole 18
    azoxystrobin 2, 8, 18
    benomyl 2, 18, 42
    Bordeaux mixture 2, 8, 46
    bupirimate 73, 74
    captan 2, 73, 74, 175
    captafol 18
    carbendazim 8, 18, 73, 157, 173, 179
    carboxim 8
    chlorothanil 8, 72
    copper hydroxide 18
    copper sulphate 1, 18
    cyprodinil 8
    dithianon 73
    dithiocarbamate 179
    epoxiconazole 72
    ethaboxam 192
    fenpropidin 72
    fenpropimorph   8
    fentin hydroxide 18
    fusiláosle 157
    iprodine 18
    lead arsenate 1

lime sulphur 1
mancozeb 8, 18, 42, 74, 179
maneb 42
metalaxyl 18
propiconazole 8
prothioconazole 192
stobilurin 192
sulphur 18
tebuconazole 8, 72
tetraconazole 18, 175
thiram 2, 18, 157
tridimefon 74
tributyltin 42
zineb 2, 42
ziram 42

Game Conservancy 153
GAP 30, 43, 168, 174, 176, 182, 204
gas chromatography 171
gel 64
generation study 31
genetically modified crops 12, 71, 184, 191,
        195, 199, 200
genotoxicity 31
gibberellin 173
GIS 138, 203
glasshouse 66, 67, 69, 127, 186
glasshouse sprayer 49
gloves 84, 85, 89, 90, 98, 100, 127, 128
glycoalkaloid 180
glucosinates 180
GM crops 12, 71, 184, 191, 195, 199, 200
GMHT 200
goggles 82
Good Agricultural Practice 30, 43, 168, 174,
        176, 182, 204
Google 2
GPS 53, 58, 139, 203
granule 3, 31, 41, 68, 124, 158, 159
granule treatment 13
Green Revolution 201
groundwater 110, 145, 156, 158
growth stage 72
GS 72

hands 84, 85, 88, 89, 90, 96, 99, 122, 125,
        126, 128

hand wash 127
harvesters 128
hat 83
head 85, 100
Health and Consumer Protection DG 30
Health and Safety Executive 29, 34, 98, 108
Health Protection Agency 109
hedge 109. 140, 147, 149
helicopter 52, 148
herbicides 5, 6, 9, 15, 18, 59, 74, 79, 86, 120,
        124, 142, 144, 145, 148, 150, 151,
        153, 154, 159, 184, 192, 197
  2,4-D 1,2, 7, 18, 42, 109
  2,4,5-T 42
  acetochlor 93
  Agent orange 22
  alachlor 42
  ametryne 18
  amitrole 42
  asulam 148
  atrazine 7, 18, 42, 115, 124, 145
  bentazone 18
  dicamba 18
  dichlorprop 18
  diflufenican 72
  diquat 23
  diuron 7, 144
  DNOC 2
  fenoxaprop-P-ethyl 72
  ferrous sulphate 2
  fluazifop-butyl 6
  flumeturon 7
  fluroxypr 72
  glufosinate 7, 18, 200
  glyphosate 2, 3, 6, 7, 65, 75, 136, 156,
      184, 200, 201
  isoproturon 7, 18, 72
  lenacil 157
  linuron 7
  MCPA 7, 18, 147
  mecoprop 2, 18
  metolachlor 192
  metribuzin 42
  metsulfuron-methyl 7, 72
  nitrofen 42
  paraquat 2, 6, 18, 23, 93, 94, 100, 147,
      151, 184

  propanil 18
  simazine 18
  sulfonylureas 192
  sulfosulfuron 142
  trifluralin 7, 18, 42
herbicide tolerant 71, 184, 200
hoe 10, 184
honey bee 40, 158, 160, 161
hood 100
hormones 42
hospitals 16
household pests 120
houses close to sprayed fields 121
human diseases
  encephalitis 125
  HIV/Aids 5, 185
  malaria 1, 195, 197
  onchocerciasis 146, 195
  west nile fever 16, 125
human health 19
hydraulic nozzles 50, 53, 54, 89, 115
hydraulic sprayers 46 *see also* sprayers

ICM 35, 187, 202
IGHRC 78
impregnation of fibres 46
indicators 24, 25
induction bowl 81, 96 *see also* low-level
        induction bowl (hopper)
infant 177
infective juveniles 196
ingestion 78
inhalation 38, 78, 84, 89, 91, 94, 96, 116,
     118, 127, 155
insect growth regulators 5, 151, 161, 193
insecticides (includes acaricides and insect
     growth regulators) 4, 9, 18, 79,
     154, 192
  acephate 18
  acetamprid 93
  aldicarb 4, 18, 42, 158, 159, 180
  aldrin 2
  alphacypermethrin 179
  amitraz 18
  avermectin 192
  azinphos methyl 18, 122
  bendiocarb 18, 160

bifenthrin 175
botanical 1, 196
bromopropylate 179
buprofezin 175
carbaryl 2, 21, 42
carbofuran 4, 18, 23
carbosulfan 18
chlordane 42
chlorfenvinphos 4, 175
chlorpyrifos 4, 18, 73, 74, 122, 123, 148,
    160, 177, 179
clothiaidin 193
cypermethrin 5, 179, 192
DDT 1, 2, 4, 11, 42, 115, 124, 125, 146,
    151, 152, 153, 162
deltamethrin 5, 18, 158, 160, 192
diazinon 2,4, 93, 123
dichlorvos 18, 124
dicofol 179
dieldrin 2, 4, 42, 152, 159, 197
diflubenzuron 2, 5, 160, 193, 197
dimethoate 18, 179
derris 1
endosulfan 22, 42, 118, 145, 153
endrin 4, 152
fenitrothion 18, 160, 180
fenoxycarb 73
fenpyroximate 73
fenthion 18, 151
fipronil 5, 18, 160, 193, 197
flonicamid 194
formetanate 18
HCH 2, 73, 115, 118
heptachlor 42
imidacloprid 2, 5, 18, 158, 159, 193
lambda cyhalothrin 18, 158, 160
lindane 42, 124
malathion 4, 18, 145, 160, 175
methamidophos 18, 22, 23, 119
methidathion 4
methomyl 18, 42, 127
methoprene 194
methoxychlor 42
methyl parathion 11
mevinphos 18
milbemectin 192
monocrotophos 4, 18, 22, 23

mycoinsecticide 196
nicotine 1, 18, 196
omethoate 179
parathion 2, 4, 18, 22, 42
permethrin 2, 5, 92, 125, 146, 192
phenothrin 18
phosphamidon 18
pirimicarb 72, 73, 158, 159, 175
profenophos 175, 179
propetamfos 93
propargite 179
pyrazoles 192
pyrethrins 1, 5, 151, 192
pyrethroids 42, 74, 75, 146, 151, 159,
    161, 192, 198
pyridalyl 194
pyriproxifen 146
resmethrin 18
rotenone 1, 18, 145, 196
spinosad 2, 18, 194
spirodiclofen 194
spiromesifen 194
tebufenozide 5, 194
teflubenzuron 160
temephos 4, 18, 146
tetradifon 179
thiamethoxam 193
thiodicarb 18
toxaphene 11, 42
triazopnos 18
trichlorphon 4, 18
triflumuron 160
insect management 186
insects
    Anthonomus grandis 11
    ants 16, 120 194
    aphids 14, 72, 73, 74, 159, 180, 199
    armyworms 12
    bee 40
    boll weevil 11, 198
    bollworm 11, 23, 74, 75, 199
    black flies 146, 195
    capsids 73
    Choristoneura fumiferana 15
    clouded drab moth 73
    cockroaches 16, 120, 122
    codling moth 14, 73, 198

collembolan 201
colorado beetle 14
fruit flies 188
gypsy moth 15
Helicoverpa armigera 11
Helicoverpa zea 11, 199
jassids 74
Leptinotarsa decemlineata 14
locusts 12, 159, 195, 197
Lymantria dispar 15
Lymantria monacha 15
mosquitoes 16, 46, 66, 124, 125, 146,
        194, 195, 197
nun moth 15
pine beauty moth 195
pink bollworm 198
psyllids 194
saw fly 73, 195
scale 194
Simulium 146
spruce budworm 15
stem borers 12
termites 120
Tortrix 73
tsetse flies 146, 198
vine weevil 5, 196
weevils 14
wheat bulb fly 152
whiteflies 74, 186, 194
integrated crop management 35, 187, 202
integrated pest management 10, 35, 43, 101,
        128, 156, 186, 187, 190, 194, 202,
        203, 204
Interdepartmental Group on Health Risks
        from Chemicals 78
International Organisation for Standardization
        (ISO) 29, 110, 112
International Rice Research Institute 10
International Union of Pure and Applied
        Chemistry 29, 33
IOBC 161
IPM 10, 35, 43, 101, 128, 156, 186, 187, 190,
        194, 202, 203, 204
IR-4 172
irritancy 31
ISO 29
IUPAC 29, 115

Jazzercize 121
juice 175
juvenile hormone analogues 194

kairomones 197
knapsack sprayer 19, 20, 44, 46, 60, 62, 63,
        83, 89, 100, 199
King Edward 180

label 43, 120, 159, 203
laser equipment 54
Latin American diet 176
laundering 79, 82
lawns 16, 120
LDL 181
leaching 143, 185
lead-free fuel 201
LEAF 187
leaf wetness 185
legislation 16
leg (s) 85, 99, 100
Leicestershire 124
'Lenape' 180
LERAP 133, 134, 135, 138, 142, 203
'Liaison' 170
Lidar 113, 148
limit of detection 93, 174, 176
limit of quantification 172
Lincolnshire 124
Linking Environment and Farming 187
lipoproteins 181
liver 179
loading 128
local authority sprayer 49
Local Environmental Risk Assessment for
        Pesticides 133, 134, 135, 138, 142, 203
lockers 98
Locustox 161
LOD 93, 174, 176
LOEL 32
long-term studies 32
LOQ 172
Lowest Observable Effect Level 32
low-level induction bowl (hopper) 81, 96
'lure and kill' 198

mammals 158, 161, 181, 201

margin of exposure 78
Maris Piper 180
mask(s) 84, 100
mating disruption 198
Mato Grosso do Sul 23
Maximum Residue Levels 17, 43, 75, 156, 168, 170, 172, 173, 174, 175, 179, 181
measurement of drift 110, 134, 135
Medical and Toxicological Panel 39
Medicines Act 108
Member States 30
mepiquat chloride 72
metabolism 31
Metarhizium anisopliae 5, 160, 162, 195
methylated vegetable oil 192
methyl bromide 114
methyl isocyanate 19
middle eastern diet 176
mineral oil 72
minimum tillage 3, 186
minnow 40
mist 56
mites 73
mixing 128
model 113, 144, 145, 155, 203
MOE 78
monitoring crops 71, 188, 203
morphine 94
morpholines 8
MRL 17, 43, 75, 156, 168, 170, 172, 173, 174, 175, 179, 181
mulch 185
multiple chemical sensitivity syndrome 25
Mutual Recognition 3
mycosis 195

National Pesticide Strategy 25, 202
National Proficiency Test Council 44
National Register of Spray Operators 25, 44
National Sprayer Testing Scheme 25, 44, 58
Naturalyte 194
NAWQA 145
NEDI 174, 176, 177
nematicide 23, 41, 124
    aldicarb 2, 23, 41, 124
nematodes 14, 159, 180

neonicotinoids 5, 193, 194
NESTI 174, 176
neutron activation analysis 112
NGO 24
NOAEL 32, 78, 89
NOEL 32
noise 85
Nolan rules 29
non-ionic wetter 72
Non-target Arthropod Regulatory Resting 41
No Observed Adverse Effect Level 32, 78
No Observed Effect Level 32
noodles 175
nose 108
no-till 185
nozzles 203
    air induction 54, 56, 57, 117, 134, 136, 144
    angling 57, 196
    colour coding 58
    cone 50, 59
    deflector 54
    even-spray 57
    flat fan 50, 54, 59, 117, 136
    low pressure 54
    pre-orifice 54
    'Raindrop' 148
    rotary atomisers 59, 69, 203
    shielded 63
    trigger operated 16
    twin fluid 56
NPTC 24, 44
NPV 195
NRoSo 25, 44
NSTS 44
nuclear magnetic resonance 25
nuclear polyhedrosis viruses 195
nuisance pests 16
number of sprays 71, 196

octanol 198
octanol-water partition 144
odour 108, 118, 198
OECD 155
oestrogenic 124
operator exposure 76, 78, 85, 86, 87, 89, 101, 156

operator proficiency 43
operator safety 203
organic 24, 180, 181, 191
organochlorine 4, 22, 94, 124, 145, 151, 152,
        153, 169, 178, 192, 197
organophosphate 4, 21, 22, 92, 94, 122, 124,
        127, 145, 146, 151, 161, 173, 177,
        194, 195
overalls *see* coveralls

PACE 142
packaging 35, 79
Paracelsus 181
paracetomol 181
partridge 153
passerines 153
patch spraying 6, 187, 197
pathways 16
PBO (piperonyl butoxide) 125
PCBs 125, 126
PEC 39, 40, 41, 156, 158, 161
peel 175
peeling 174, 175, 176
pEMA 156
Pentland Hawk 180
peregrine falcon 152
perma-net 124
persistence 151, 152, 169
personal protective equipment 4, 16, 35, 68,
        83, 91, 93
Pesticide Action Network 24, 201
pesticide application equipment 23
pesticide classification 17
pesticide exposure 25
Pesticide Forum 155
Pesticide Handlers Exposure Database 79
Pesticide Incidents Appraisal Panel 25, 108
Pesticide Initiative Programme 174
pesticide residues 24, 25
Pesticide Residue Committee 170, 179
Pesticide Risk Assessment Peer Review 30
Pesticide Safety Directorate 2, 34
Pesticide Safety Precaution Scheme 16
Petri dish 112
PHED 79, 88
phenoxy herbicides 7
phenylpyrazole 5

pheromones 197
pheromone trapping 186, 189
phosphono-amino acids 7
pheasant 153
PHI 75, 168, 172, 178
PIAP 25, 108
PIC 17
PIP 174, 178
plant breeding 187
plant diseases
    blight 14, 180
    Botrytis 75
    canker 73
    fusarium 14
    mildew 14, 72, 73, 74
    scab 14, 73, 74
    Sigatoka 14
    Septoria 72
plant growth regulator 72
plant vigour 40
PM10 201
point source 143
poison centre 95
pollination 40
polyphenols 181
polypropylene 79
polythene line 112
pomace 175
POP 155
potential toxicity 31
PPE 4, 16, 35, 68, 83, 91, 93, 99, 115, 203
PRC 170, 179
Precautionary Measures against Toxic
        Chemicals 29
predatory birds 8
Predicted Environmental Concentration 40
pre-harvest interval 75, 168, 172, 178
pressure packs 46, 64, 120, 123
PRG 161
Prior Informed Consent 17
probabilistic model(ling) 25, 148, 178
processing samples 171
procyanidins 181
product label 25
prophylactic treatment 69
protected cropping 126
protective clothing 4, 16, 35, 68, 83, 115

PSD 2, 34, 119
ptaquiloside 145
puffer packs 62
pulp 175
pyrethroid(s) 5, 42, 74, 75, 124, 146, 151, 159, 161, 192, 198

quail 40
Quelea 151

rabbits 31
RAC 174, 175
railway 144
rain 110, 115, 143, 144, 159, 184, 185
rats 31, 42
raw agricultural produce 174, 175
red fescue 155
registration of pesticides 29, 203, 204
REI 127
reptiles 160, 161
residents 25, 115, 119, 120
Residue Committee 170
residues 30, 32, 40, 101, 120, 146, 156, 169, 173, 174, 175, 176, 178, 179, 181, 182
residues in food 168
resistance management 185
respirator 68, 84, 92
restaurants 16
restricted entry intervals 127
retailers 178
rinsing containers 81
risk assessment 31, 69, 110, 124, 128, 158, 174, 179
risk information 157
risk indicator 158
risk quotient 41
river 110, 143
roads 143, 144
roadshow 25
rodenticides 8, 18, 180
    brodifacoum 18
    bromadiolone 8
    difenacoum 8
    warfarin 8, 18
roses 16
rotary atomisers 59, 60, 69

rotary samplers 113
rotorods 113
Royal Commission on Environmental Pollution 25, 30, 108, 119
Royal Society for the Protection of Birds 151
RPE 68, 84, 92
rule of nines 87, 88
'run-off' 142, 143, 159

sachets 35, 44, 84
safener 69
samplers 112
scouting 71, 187, 188
sedimentation data 110
seeds 154, 187
seed germination 40
seed treatment 69, 74, 186, 196
selective application 196
sensitivity of individuals 119
set-aside 65, 129
sheep dip 90, 92, 145
shelf life 182
shrimp 40
Single Farm Payment 129
skin 78, 82, 89, 92, 122, 125, 198
skin wipes 127
slugs 180
socks 98
soil 146, 156, 159, 184, 185, 202
solanine 180
solenoid valve 58
space treatment 66
sparrowhawks 152
spawning 40
spillage 143
spray classification 54, 55
spray concentration 75
spray drift 54, 56, 108, 133, 143, 147, 148, 150, 196, 203
sprayers 23
    air-blast 95, 156
    compression 46, 59, 61, 124
    glasshouse 49
    knapsack 19, 20, 44, 46, 60, 62, 63, 83, 89, 100, 199
    lever-operated 60, 62

local authority 49
mistblower 62
orchard 140
self-propelled 48
tractor-mounted 48, 89, 95, 116, 140
trailed 48, 150
trigger-operated 65, 120
trolley mounted 99
tunnel 88, 138, 140, 141, 203
turf 49
sprayer testing 58
sprayer washing 101, 144, 203
spray operators 43, 202
spray preparation 95
spray quality 58, 59
spray spectra 54
spray tracer 112
spray volume 47, 59, 75, 89, 98, 128, 168
spot treatment 129, 197
standards 23, 174
Statutory Codes of Practice 17
stenching agent 23
stewardship 23, 25
STMR 176
stobilurins 8
storage 70
strip cropping 151
structural pest control 120
substituted ureas 7
suicide 22, 23, 34, 92, 181
sulfonylureas 7
surface run-off 110
surface tension 136
supermarket 173
swabs 88
SWATCATCH 145
syndrome 25

table tennis balls 112
tablets 44
tax 25, 144, 148
TCDD 22
teachers 124
TER 40, 41
teratogenicity 31
thematic strategy 24

thermal fogger 66, 67, 68, 125
thigh 100
thyroid 179
tillage 15, 184, 201
timber 124
time-weighted average 128
time-weighted sample 114
timing of sprays 71, 196
timothy grass 155
TMDI 174, 175, 176
tobacco smoke 38
toddler 177
torso 100
Toxic and Persistent Substances Centre 145
toxicity exposure ratio 40
toys 122
tractor cab 93, 98
training 35
transfer factor 174, 175
translaminar 75
triazines 7
triazoles 8
Trichogramma 186
triple rinse 96
trout 40
turbulence 138
turf 144
turf sprayer 49
TWA 128
'twist-tie' 198

ultra-violet light 87, 195
ULV 59, 75, 101
underwear 98
uncertainty factor 32, 78
urban 16, 142
urea 73, 74
urine 92, 93

vapour 108
vapour drift 109
vector control 16, 46, 124
vegetable oil 192
vegetation 147, 150, 151
vehicle exhausts 38, 201
vehicle mounted equipment 16

veterinary medicines 29
VLV 59, 101
volatile 114
volatile organic content (VOC) 118
volatilisation 143, 155
Voluntary Initiative 24, 25, 59, 155, 159
vultures 153

washing hands 82
waste management 43, 203
waste regulations 101
water 25, 40, 133, 142, 143, 145, 147
watercourses 133, 136, 139, 159, 196
water tank 84, 98, 110, 143
weaver birds 151
weeds 72, 74, 129, 153, 154, 187, 196, 200
   blackgrass 72
   charlock 72
   cleavers 72
   poppies 72
   ragged robin 147
   Striga 12
weed competition 9
weeding 9, 12
weed management 184
Weed Society of America 6

weed wiper 65, 66, 197
'weevil sticks' 198
weight measurements 32
WHO 17, 19, 22, 34, 78, 101, 124, 125, 173,
   174, 175, 199
wildflowers 154
'wildlife strips' 154
wind breaks 140, 148
wind direction 140
wind speed 112, 149
wind speed checking 137
wind tunnel 112, 113, 136
wine 181
woodland 150, 153
World Health Organisation 17, 19, 22, 34, 78,
   101, 124, 125, 173, 174, 175, 199
worker exposure 108, 115, 126, 127
worker protection standards 127
world sales of pesticides 3

xenobiotics 180, 181

yellowhammer 153

zero tillage 3, 184
Zuckerman 29